Infectious Diseases

Barbara A. Bannister

BSc, LRCP MRCS,
MB BS, MRCP(UK)

Lecturer in Medical Microbiology
St Bartholomew's Hospital,
West Smithfield, London, EC1

Formerly Senior Registrar in Infectious Diseases
The Royal Free Hospital, Coppetts Wood Hospital,
Muswell Hill, London, N10 1JN

Baillière Tindall · London

Published by Baillière Tindall,
1 St Anne's Road, Eastbourne, East Sussex BN21 3UN

© 1983 Baillière Tindall

First published 1983

ISBN 0 7020 1009 X

Typeset by Bookens, Saffron Walden, Essex
Printed in Great Britain by
Garden City Press, Letchworth, Herts

British Library Cataloguing in Publication Data

Bannister, Barbara A.
  Infectious diseases.—(Concise Medical Textbook)
  1. Communicable diseases
  I. Title
  616.9   RC111
  ISBN 0-7020-1009-X

Contents

Preface

The science, or art, of medicine is best learnt by experience. This truth is well-recognized by students at all stages of their careers, who often travel many miles to attend practical and clinical teaching courses. In no specialty is the need for such experience greater than in infectious diseases, for these can strike at any or all of the body systems in patients whose ages range from the moment of birth to the extremes of longevity.

In addition to this, the increasing use of immunosuppressive therapy has produced a new range of opportunistic infections which present testing diagnostic problems. Nowadays a physician can be expected to distinguish between this wide variety of infectious conditions, toxic conditions, allergy and autoimmune disease. A surgeon, similarly, must be aware of the range of infections which can mimic, or even cause, acute surgical disorders.

This book is designed to provide the broad background of infectious diseases learning which is required in modern medical practice. As well as the conventional enumeration of infectious conditions and their management, each chapter has an initial discussion section in which the infections are considered in the context of their presenting features and their overlap with other medical and surgical conditions. Particular attention is paid to differential diagnosis as an active sequence of events. The avoidance of common diagnostic pitfalls is emphasized, as is the importance of checking the patient's progress both during and after treatment.

The systematic presentation of the chapters is based on the clinical teaching offered to medical students of the Royal Free Hospital School of Medicine. It also includes material used in the Joint Board of Clinical Nursing Studies course for specialist infectious diseases nurses, and in the Whittington Hospital course for the first part of the examination for Membership of the Royal College of Physicians.

The emphasis on the clinical approach to infection is reinforced by a ready-reference section on antibiotic usage and dosage to be found at the end of each clinical chapter. This is intended for on-the-spot use, and is not a substitute for a textbook of antimicrobial chemotherapy. Most of the recommended dosages are the same as those found in the *British National Formulary*. Differences sometimes occur in emergency situations, when very high doses of non-toxic drugs such as penicillin are given in an effort to achieve high tissue or cerebrospinal fluid drug levels without delay.

The purpose of the book is twofold. Firstly, it is intended to provide a learning text for medical students and specialist nurses, and to help in preparation for their qualifying examinations. Secondly, it is designed as a bedside aid to the diagnosis and management of infectious diseases, for use by medical students, busy house officers and general practitioners. It also contains information on subjects which often feature in MRCP Part I questions, and on matters of interest to Community Medicine trainees.

It is not possible for a concise textbook to encompass the whole universe of infection, including specialist discussion of subjects such as epidemiology, or immunology or the rarer tropical diseases. For more comprehensive information the reader is recommended to consult some of the excellent reference books available for further study.

I sincerely hope that this book will be a trusty companion to many medical students and other students of infectious diseases, and that it will not desert them when they set out on their clinical careers.

February 1983   B. A. BANNISTER

Acknowledgements

I welcome the opportunity to thank the many people whose generosity and encouragement have supported the production of this book. Their contributions of labour and material have both enhanced the text and delivered the author from the occasional threat of despair.

The Director and the Staff of the Communicable Diseases Surveillance Centre have supplied much of the epidemiological data, and have provided figures 21, 22, 23b and 26.

Statistics on air travel were provided by the Civil Aviation Authority Statistics Unit.

The Public Health Laboratory Service Malaria Reference Laboratory at the Ross Institute at the London School of Hygiene and Tropical Medicine provided the map which is reproduced in Figure 25.

Mrs Margaret Bannister far exceeded all maternal obligations in volunteering to cope with the great volume of typing, and bore the resulting hardships with characteristic good humour. Additional help was kindly given by Mrs Rosemary Smith and Mrs Betty Inman.

Finally, and most importantly, I am indebted to my two editors Mrs Ann Saadi and Mr Graham Smith, not only for their unflagging support and attention to detail, but also for never losing their sense of humour. Their many suggestions and practical hints, as well as their valuable criticism, have greatly added to the quality of the completed book.

1

Concepts of Infectious Diseases and their Management

'Infection' is the result of invasion of the body by micro-organisms which cause damage to its tissues. 'Communicable disease' indicates that the infection is contracted by contact with a source of micro-organisms.

Sources of infection

Micro-organisms are everywhere. They colonize man, animals, food, water and soil, and human infection can be acquired from any of these sources. A summary of some common modes of spread of infection is given in Table 1.

Body defences against infection

Surface barriers.   Before it can cause an infection, the pathogenic agent must be able to penetrate the surface of the host by passing through the skin or mucous membranes. The keratinous surface of the skin and its layered structure make it very resistant to penetration unless there is an open wound exposing the subcutaneous tissues. The mucous membranes, however, are much more delicate and may be penetrated even when intact. The mucosae of the respiratory, urinary and alimentary tracts are common points of entry for pathogens.

Secretions.   Tears, urine and mucus tend to wash organisms away from mucosal surfaces, and propel them to the exterior. In addition, secretions contain lysozymes, acids and antibodies which attack organisms and reduce the surface load of potential pathogens.

The normal body flora.   Most skin and mucosal surfaces are occupied by a variety of organisms which cause no harm to the host tissues (Table 2). These not only occupy the available space, but some of them also produce substances which make the environment unfavourable to intruders. In this way the establishment of pathogenic organisms is discouraged. Normal flora is only harmless when confined to body surfaces. If surface organisms enter the tissues or circulation, however, they are quite capable of causing serious disease.

It can be seen that defects in skin or mucosal surfaces, failure of se-

Table 1.   Examples of spread of infection from various sources

Method of spread	Comments	Examples
Air currents	Viruses adhere to dust or moisture particles, and can therefore be trapped by high efficiency particular (HEPA) filters, as can bacteria and spores	Chickenpox, anthrax, nocardiosis
Droplet spread	During coughing and sneezing	Influenza, whooping cough
Aerosol	Domestic and industrial water; laboratory specimens during pipetting or centrifugation	Legionnaire's disease, tuberculosis
Water	By contact with mucosa or broken skin; pathogen bores through skin	Leptospirosis, schistosomiasis, strongyloidiasis
Direct contact	From animal or human skin	Impetigo, ringworm, scabies
Soil	Entry via skin lesion	Tetanus, gas gangrene
Faecal–oral	Hand-to-mouth; sewage-contaminated food or water	Gastroenteritis, enteric fevers, gut helminths and protozoa
Inoculation	By tooth, claw or needle	*Pasteurella multocida*, cat scratch disease, hepatitis B
Vector	Inoculation by the bite of a sucking arthropod which is also a host.	Yellow fever, malaria, typhus

cretions or alteration of the normal flora due to a change in the environment, or to antibiotic administration, will leave the host poorly defended against surface attack.

Tissue and bloodstream defence
The tissue fluid and bloodstream contain cells and proteins which can attack invading organisms before the immune response is mounted.

Phagocytes.   The granulocyte and macrophage series of cells can ingest foreign particles, bacteria and debris. They secrete proteases, catalases and other lysozymes which attack particles both inside and outside the cell. They also initiate the activity of kinins and taxins which enhance inflammation and attract further phagocytes. The activation of the phagocyte's cell surface initiates the production of prostaglandins.

Eosinophils.   These are cells of the granulocyte series which have a special affinity for allergic and anaphylactic reactions. They play a vital part in the body's defences against parasitic infections.

Table 2. Some normal flora of the human body

Skin
 Staphylococci
 Streptococcus pyogenes
 Corynebacteria (several species)
 Candida spp.
Conjunctiva
 Staphylococci
 Corynebacteria
Nasopharynx
 Haemophilus influenzae
 Streptococcus pneumoniae
 Microaerophilic streptococci
 Anaerobic bacilli
Mouth and throat
 Many viridans streptococci
 Streptococcus pyogenes
 Streptococcus pneumoniae
 Haemophilus influenzae
 Neisseria spp.
 Anaerobic bacilli
 Candida albicans
 Spirochaetes
 Actinomyces spp.

Small bowel merging into
 Lactobacilli
 Escherichia coli
 Candida albicans

       Large bowel
       Microaerophilic streptococci
       Faecal streptococci
       Bacteroides and *Clostridium* spp.
       Candida albicans
       Protozoa
       Bifidobacterium and Eubacterium

Female genital tract
 Lactobacilli
 Coliform bacilli
 Group B streptococci
 Faecal streptococci
 Bacteroides and *Clostridium* species
 Candida albicans
 Ureaplasmas
Areas usually without normal flora
 Stomach
 Pancreaticobiliary tract
 Pulmonary alveoli
 Urinary tract

The alternative complement pathway. This involves the activation of the complement system directly by substances in bacterial capsules or cell membranes, and results in lysis of the organisms. The importance of this defence is suggested by the increased incidence of severe infections in some families and individuals who lack complement components. Lack of the complement component C3 is associated with a lack of bacteriocidal activity in the blood, while lack of C5, C6, C7 and C8 predisposes to severe infection with Gram-negative cocci.

Humoral immunity.   On exposure to pathogens in the host's tissues or bloodstream, B-lymphocytes become active, and develop into immunoglobulin-secreting plasma cells. There are several classes of immunoglobulin, but the first to appear is IgM. This is a large polyvalent molecule which can take part in agglutination reactions with antigen, and can also fix complement to initiate cell lysis via the classical complement pathway. IgM is later gradually replaced by IgG, which is the main circulating antibody. Once IgG production is established, a further exposure to the same antigen will result in a sudden large increase in IgG antibody, the so-called secondary response. Like IgM, IgG fixes complement. IgG is a smaller molecule, and can cross the normal placenta.

Two other immunoglobulins take part in the immune responses. The main secreted immunoglobulin is IgA, present in tears, saliva, colostrum and mucosal secretions. It does not fix complement, but it coats surface pathogens, making them more easily phagocytosed and reducing their ability to adhere to surfaces. IgE exists mainly bound to cells, particularly to mast cells. On combination with antigen it causes the mast cells to degranulate, releasing histamine and other kinins.

Defects of production of one or more immunoglobulins due to congenital or acquired conditions renders an individual susceptible to bacterial disease, as circulating pathogens cannot be effectively attacked in the absence of circulating factors. Even the non-specific defence afforded by phagocytes is less efficient in the absence of antibody.

Cell-mediated immunity.   This involves the destruction of infected cells, or large pathogens such as yeasts and fungi, by a system of T-lymphocytes. Cytotoxic, or killer, cells destroy cells bearing the antigen to which they are sensitized. Helper cells enhance antibody secretion by plasma cells, and suppressor cells modulate T-lymphocyte activity, probably in order to prevent destructive overactivity of the immune response.

Defects of cell-mediated immunity leave the individual susceptible to viral and fungal infections. A few cases of severe combined immunodeficiency (SCID) are described, who have little resistance to any kind of infection. Immune deficiencies are increasingly often due to treatment with corticosteroids and cytotoxic drugs. Malignant disease of the bone marrow or other reticuloendothelial tissues can also cause loss of humoral or cellular immunity.

The spleen.   Damaged, dead and infected cells, together with bacteria and other particles, are removed from the circulation by the spleen. There is also evidence that the spleen produces humoral factors which modulate the activities of lymphocytes. Loss of splenic function makes the individual more susceptible to severe bacterial infection, particularly pneumococcal septicaemia.

Other factors influencing resistance to infection
Many systems are known to affect, or possibly to take part in, the body's response to infection. Such factors as the patient's HLA type, endocrine status, metabolic rate and state of nutrition can all influence the likelihood or severity of infection. Recent exposure to metabolic stress or another infection may impair phagocytosis and the immune response. This may explain, for instance, the association between viral respiratory infections and subsequent bacterial bronchopneumonia.

The result of exposure to infection therefore depends on the patient's general health and the completeness of his body defences, together with the virulence of the organism, the tissue damage it causes, the tissue damage resulting from toxin release and cell destruction during the immune response, and the patient's previous exposure to present and other pathogens. All of these factors must be borne in mind throughout the process of diagnosis and management of infectious diseases.

Fever

A stable body temperature is maintained by the action of the hypothalamus on the autonomic nervous system. The oral temperature varies between 35.8 °C and 37 °C with a tendency to the higher level in late evening. The rectal temperature is about 0.5 °C above the oral and the axillary temperature is about 0.2 °C below it.

During a feverish response macrophages are activated by foreign antigens or the products of immune reactions. They produce a low molecular weight protein, leukocytic pyrogen, which acts on the hypothalamus to reset the temperature level.

Consequences of fever
The advantages of a fever are debatable. It is true that a higher temperature may not favour the existence of some pathogens, but it may equally be an encouragement to others. In some infections cold agglutinins or haemolysins are produced and a raised temperature may afford protection from their effects, but this is an uncommon situation. There are several disadvantages of fever which cause considerable problems in patient care. A raised temperature imposes a proportionate rise in metabolic rate so that the pulse rate rises by about 20 beats per minute for every 1 °C rise in temperature. Any tendency to catabolism is therefore greatly increased by fever.

Rigors.   These are uncontrollable shaking attacks which may last for only a few moments or up to an hour. They are usually associated with a rapidly rising temperature during bacteraemia. They cause severe physical and mental distress to the patient and greatly increase the metabolic output.

Convulsions.   Children aged between 1 and 6 years, as well as patients with epilepsy, sometimes have fits during episodes of fever. If the fever persists it may be necessary to give anticonvulsants temporarily to avoid injury or exhaustion.

A small oral or intramuscular dose of diazepam may be sufficient, but if intravenous diazepam is used to terminate convulsions great care must be taken not to induce respiratory arrest, especially in children. For use over a number of days, oral phenytoin 25–50 mg once or twice daily for children, and 100–300 mg daily for adults, is probably most effective, though it is not always the drug of choice for long-term prophylaxis in children. For adults with intractable fits chlormethiazole (Heminevrin) 0.8% infusion 40–100 ml initially may be effective, and is then titrated to produce light sleep. Respiratory depression is sometimes a problem with this drug.

Delirium.   This may occur in the young, the old or those with a very high fever (41 °C or more). Urinary retention commonly accompanies delirium, and injury may result from restless or aggressive movement. The use of sedatives rarely has more than a transient effect, and often only makes the patient more confused and restless. Relief of pain and of urinary retention, with avoidance of irritating restraint, is usually the best course, as the undisturbed patient will often rest for short periods of time.

Reducing the patient's temperature
A temporary reduction of 1 or 2 °C in body temperature can be obtained by bathing or sponging the skin with tepid water. The effect can be prolonged by fanning. Several litres of fluid may be lost daily in sweat, and sufficient water and electrolyte replacement should be provided by the oral or intravenous route.

Antipyretic drugs.   These may be used if simple measures are not effective. The best is aspirin 600 mg up to 4-hourly (50 mg/kg daily in divided doses for infants and children). Some units use paracetamol 1 g up to 4-hourly (120 mg four times daily for infants; 240–500 mg four times daily for children over age 2).

Many of the unwanted effects of fever can be ameliorated or avoided by attention to simple methods of temperature reduction.

Diagnostic methods

History

Exposure. The clinical history provides vital information on exposure to the sources of infection mentioned in Table 1. Special enquiry should be made about exposure at work, during travel abroad and during visits to restaurants and resorts. Domestic pets may also be a source of infection, as may animals, birds or insects encountered during holidays.

Incubation. The time between exposure and illness may correspond to the incubation period of a particular disease, or it may exclude that disease by exceeding the possible incubation period. It is therefore important to determine the dates of exposure and of first symptoms of disease.

Immunity. It is important also to determine the immune status of the patient, as a previous attack, or immunization, may help to exclude some diseases from the differential diagnosis.

Symptoms and signs. The evolution of many diseases is characteristic, so that the order of appearance of fever, diarrhoea, rash, etc. should be established as definitely as possible.

Previous treatment. Finally it should be remembered that concurrent antibiotic treatment may alter a disease without curing it, and will certainly affect the result of bacteriological cultures. Treatment with corticosteroids or cytotoxic agents should be enquired for, as this will affect the ultimate prognosis.

Physical examination
During the examination of the patient it is particularly helpful to note the mental state, as some infections are often associated with exhaustion, confusion, irritation or coma.

Inflammatory lesions. The site of inflammatory lesions is important, so that the tonsils, tympanic membranes, conjunctivae and perineum should not be neglected if examination is to be complete. The distribution of lymph node enlargement and involvement of the liver or spleen should also be noted.

Rashes (Fig.1). The presence of a typical rash is a very helpful aid to diagnosis, though it should be remembered that many rashes are not caused by infections. Poisoning, allergy, malignancy and metabolic disorders may be associated with rashes which resemble those of infectious diseases. The whole skin surface should be examined for signs of a rash

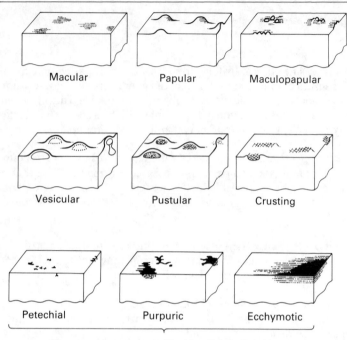

Macular   Papular   Maculopapular

Vesicular   Pustular   Crusting

Petechial   Purpuric   Ecchymotic

These rashes are caused by bleeding in the skin.
They do not blanch on pressure

Fig. 1. Diagrammatic description of types of rashes.

(exanthem) and mucosal surfaces should not be neglected as certain diseases also produce an internal rash (enanthem). The presence of even a single typical lesion in such diseases as enteric fever, meningococcal or gonococcal septicaemia, or syphilis may allow prompt diagnosis and immediate treatment.

Urine testing.   Ward testing of the urine should be part of the initial assessment of the patient, as it may give vital information for diagnosis and prognosis. The presence of bile in the urine may allow the diagnosis of hepatitis to be made, while the presence of blood after an attack of streptococcal tonsillitis could indicate nephritis.

Repeated examination.   Because infectious diseases evolve over hours, days or weeks, it is essential to examine the patient several times until the diagnosis is clear, and during treatment and follow-up. If this is not done, fluctuations of consciousness, fleeting rashes or changing heart murmurs may be missed, and the prompt diagnosis and management of the disease will be delayed unnecessarily.

Notes on the use of antibiotics

Antibiotics are antimicrobial substances naturally produced by micro-organisms. Although an increasing number of antimicrobial drugs are now prepared synthetically, the term antibiotic is often loosely applied to all of such drugs, and will be so used in this book.

Antibiotics are potent and potentially dangerous drugs which always have unwanted effects on the patient, and often on the patient's environment as well. Side-effects of antibiotics include nausea, vomiting, diarrhoea, colitis, fever, rash, deafness, jaundice, exfoliative dermatitis, nephritis, renal failure and bone marrow depression. The patient's normal body flora is always altered by antibiotic treatment, with the wider spectrum drugs producing the most severe effects. As the patient acquires an increasingly antibiotic-resistant flora this may spread to both his contacts and his environment, leading to the existence of a population of highly resistant organisms. Hospital wards are easily affected by this process. For these reasons antibiotics should be used as sparingly as possible, consistent with adequate treatment of the patient, and the drug with the narrowest spectrum of activity which includes the 'target' organisms should be the drug of choice.

Situations in which antibiotics are inappropriate
Viral infections.   No viral infection will be favourably influenced by antibiotic therapy. This tenet applies to the vast majority of upper respiratory infections, sore throats and childhood diseases in particular. Although it is a counsel of perfection never to treat such infections speculatively with antibiotics, it is possible in many situations to adopt a policy of symptomatic treatment, and a prompt 'cure' often follows.

Bacterial infections.   It is also true that some bacterial infections are not responsive to antibiotic therapy. A common example of this is intestinal infection which often resolves most quickly if treated by symptomatic measures alone.

Predisposing factors.   Certain bacterial infections cannot be abolished by antibiotic treatment because of a predisposing factor, such as stagnation in an obstructed kidney or gall bladder, tissue ischaemia in bedsores or varicose ulcers, and persisting abscesses after abdominal sepsis. In such situations bacteriological cure is often not possible, even with 'appropriate' antibiotic therapy, until the predisposing factor has been treated.

Choice of antibiotics
This should be based on the physician's knowledge of the disease and organisms, combined with the results of sensitivity tests done in the laboratory. Sometimes treatment can be firmly decided on clinical

grounds alone. Occasionally a drug will be ineffective *in vivo* when *in vitro* tests suggest otherwise. Always ask the patient if he has a history of allergy to antibiotics before commencing therapy. A second allergic reaction is often worse than the first.

Route of administration
In general orally administered therapy is adequate for superficial skin infections, mild chest infections and urinary tract infections, while parenteral therapy is required for severe parenchymal infections. Septicaemia, meningitis and endocarditis usually demand high dose intravenous therapy.

Chloramphenicol, fusidic acid and clindamycin are exceptions to this rule as they are so well absorbed by the gut that they can be given orally in almost any situation, provided that the patient is able to swallow and absorb them.

Unsuccessful antibiotic therapy
If the patient has not responded to treatment after the expected time, the situation should be reassessed. It is unwise to add further antibiotics to the regimen as the patient is more likely to end by being poisoned than by being cured. If possible it is best to stop treatment, repeat cultures and start afresh. The diagnosis should be reviewed; the cultures and sensitivity tests should be checked; and consideration should be given to the route of administration and dose of the drug, both of which may have been inappropriate.

Communicable disease surveillance in Britain

Local matters
In Britain every local authority designates a 'proper officer' who receives information concerning infection in the community. This officer is the Medical Officer of Environmental Health (MOEH) or his appointed deputy, whose duty it is to investigate and control the local situation. The MOEH has powers which enable him to ask people to be examined, to remain away from work or to provide specimens for investigation. He has few powers to compel cooperation, though failure to fulfil his request can be an offence against the various Health Services and Public Health Acts, a circumstance which adds to the MOEH's persuasion. He may particularly request food, dairy or slaughterhouse workers and school or nursery teachers to refrain from working until they are no longer infectious, and arrange for them to be compensated for loss of earnings by the Local Authority.

Statutory notification
It is statutorily required of an attending physician in Britain that he notifies all cases or *suspected* cases of designated diseases in writing to the MOEH (Table 3). The Authority provides forms for this purpose. In

Table 3.   Statutorily notifiable diseases

England, Wales and Scotland
Anthrax
Cholera
Diphtheria
Dysentery
Acute encephalitis
   infective
   postinfectious
Food poisoning
Infective jaundice
Lassa fever
†Leptospirosis
Malaria
Marburg disease
Measles
Acute meningitis
Ophthalmia neonatorum
Paratyphoid fever
Plague
Acute poliomyelitis
   paralytic
   non-paralytic
Rabies
†Relapsing fever
Scarlet fever
Smallpox
†Tetanus
Tuberculosis (all forms)
Typhoid fever
Typhus fever
Viral haemorrhagic diseases
Whooping cough
†Yellow fever

Additionally notifiable in Scotland
Chicken pox
Continued fever
Encephalitis lethargica
Erysipelas
Paratyphoid fever A and B
Pneumonia (acute influenzal)
Pneumonia (acute primary)
*Pneumonia (not otherwise notifiable)
Puerperal fever
Puerperal pyrexia

*in some areas
†not notifiable in Scotland
Medical Officers of Environmental Health (MOEH) may require additional diseases to be
notified in their District.

addition to the currently notifiable diseases a MOEH may require further diseases to be notified in his area.

The MOEH is required to provide regular returns of notifications to the Office of Population Censuses and Surveys (OPCS), and to notify the Director of the Communicable Diseases Surveillance Centre of certain diseases including dangerous virus infections, and of any large or serious outbreak of infection in the District.

Communicable Diseases Surveillance Centre (CDSC)
This centre receives weekly reports of positive diagnoses on a voluntary basis, from hospital and Public Health Laboratories, individual physicians and other sources in England, Wales and Northern Ireland. It produces a weekly report, the *Communicable Diseases Report (CDR)* which is circulated in confidence to interested parties, including Specialists in Community Medicine. CDSC and OPCS jointly produce an annual report on communicable disease statistics. In Scotland the CDS report *(Communicable Diseases—Scotland)* is produced weekly.

As well as providing early warning of local and national outbreaks, and liaison with the health authorities in other countries and the World Health Organization, this system allows research and development in the fields of epidemiology and public health. In addition CDSC has an obligation to provide information and advice on the investigation and control of outbreaks, and can also send trained epidemiologists if required. Specialist training is provided for interested personnel working in Community Medicine.

Communicable disease surveillance in the United States of America
In the United States there is a system of State Epidemiologists, who report notifiable diseases weekly by telegraph to the Centers for Disease Control (CDC) Atlanta, Georgia. Other matters of interest are reported informally by epidemiologists, physicians and others. Provisional weekly statistics and comment are prepared by CDC for publication by the US Department of Health and Human Services/Public Health Service in the *Morbidity and Mortality Weekly Report (MMWR)*. The *MMWR* also contains mortality data reported voluntarily by city departments.

In addition to statistical information, CDC can offer laboratory facilities, epidemiological expertise and manpower to assist in the investigation of communicable and other disease.

Communicable disease surveillance in other countries
Departments and Ministries of Health in many countries collect information about communicable diseases and their epidemiology. Most produce frequent up-to-date reports. Other reports in English include:

1. *Canada Diseases Weekly Report* (Health and Welfare, Canada).
2. *CAREC Surveillance Report* of the Caribbean Epidemiology Centre

(Pan-American Health Organization branch of the World Health Organization).

3. *Communicable Disease Intelligence* (Environmental Health Branch, Department of Health, Australia).

The World Health Organization
This is a specialized agency of the United Nations Organization, based in Geneva, Switzerland. It carries out surveillance, investigation, immunization and eradication programmes in many countries. It aims to promote adequate health care, public services and standards of living worldwide. It also plays a part in administration of the International Health Regulations which concern the control of disease in endemic areas, and precautions to be taken by travellers.

Its reports and publications include:

1. *Weekly Epidemiological Record* (a report on disease, and progress in health care in the United Nations).
2. *World Health Bulletin.*
3. *World Health Forum.*
4. Various monthly, quarterly and annual reports.
5. Occasional reports.
6. *Health Advice to Travellers* (revised annually).

2

Skin and Mucous Membrane Infections

Introduction
A wide variety of pathogens can infect the skin and mucous membranes.
These include body flora, organisms from the air, from other people, or
from animals. The common methods of transmission are airborne or
waterborne (including by towels) or by direct contact.

Some skin eruptions are due to allergic vasculitis, in others the lesions
contain infective organisms which can be shed if the epidermal surface is
broken. Infectious rashes include those of chickenpox, herpes simplex,
syphilis and gonorrhoea.

Infective skin lesions must be distinguished from allergic or neoplastic
conditions, which can closely mimic infections or coexist with them.

Caution. The use of topical or systemic corticosteroids will often make
surface infections much worse and may lead to disastrous scarring of skin
or cornea. Indiscriminate use of corticosteroids may be regarded as
negligent in some circumstances (for example, in herpes simplex infections of the cornea).

Topical antibiotic and antihistamine preparations are potent skin sen-
sitizers, and may cause eruptions which confuse diagnosis and management. In most situations their use on the skin should be avoided.

Diagnostic methods
In some situations clinical diagnosis is possible, perhaps supplemented by
simple tests such as illumination with an ultraviolet (Woods) lamp. Light
microscopy may afford rapid diagnosis in some cases, particularly of
fungal infection.

Swabs for laboratory culture will often help to make a microbiological
diagnosis. However, a few skin flakes scraped off with a blunt scalpel are
preferable for fungal culture.

Occasionally, especially in doubtful cases, microscopy or culture of
biopsy specimens becomes necessary, and may solve a difficult
problem.

Caution. Syphilis can mimic many skin rashes. If in doubt check the
patient's serological tests for syphilis.

Warts

Epidemiology

Warts are small tumours of the skin, caused by virus infection. Different viruses are associated with simple warts, genital warts and molluscum contagiosum. Spread is by skin contact, such as holding hands, or by towels and water, especially in swimming pools or baths.

Clinical features

Simple warts. These are keratinous, well-defined swellings often on the hands or feet. They may be rather flat (plane warts) on the face or backs of hands. On the feet (plantar warts) they are pressed into the dermis by the body weight. They tend to heal after several weeks or months.

Genital warts (papillomata acuminata). These are cauliflower-like and appear on anal or genital mucosae. They often become worse during pregnancy. They must be distinguished from the flat, greasy papillomata lata of secondary syphilis, which may be accompanied by other features of syphilis (the scar of a chancre, widespread lymphadenopathy, mucous patches or snail-track ulcers in the mouth, and copper-coloured maculopapular rash extending to the palms and soles).

Molluscum contagiosum. This appears as a group of small bead-like growths, each with a central dimple. These warts may persist for months if untreated.

Diagnosis

This is almost always based on clinical findings. Rarely, biopsy may be indicated.

Treatment

Simple warts will eventually resolve if untreated; however, they can be painted or soaked with 10% formalin, or frozen with liquid nitrogen or carbon dioxide snow. They can also be curetted under local anaesthesia.

Genital warts are painted weekly with 25% podophyllin in spirit, which is washed off after 6 hours. This should not be done during pregnancy, and should be confined to external mucosae only.

Molluscum contagiosum is treated by scraping out the soft contents, or by piercing the dimple with an orangestick dipped in phenol or tincture of iodine.

Herpes simplex

Epidemiology
Herpesvirus hominis is a DNA virus which has two distinct serotypes. Type 2 is usually associated with genital infections, while other infections are mostly associated with type 1. In common with other herpes-like viruses (varicella zoster, Epstein–Barr, cytomegalovirus (CMV)), herpes simplex has the property of latency. After a more extensive primary infection, inactive virus exists in the tissues and may re-emerge to produce recurrent local lesions. Primary infection is acquired by contact, or by close-range droplet infection.

Clinical features
Primary herpetic stomatitis. This represents the response to initial infection, usually occurring in infants but occasionally in older children or young adults. There is a mildly feverish illness with tender enlargement of local lymph nodes. Many painful, shallow ulcers appear on the tongue, lips and buccal mucosa (Fig. 2). Eating may be impossible for 2 or 3 days until healing begins.

Primary genital herpes. This is similar to stomatitis, and affects the vulvovaginal or penile mucosa. Occasionally there is interference with sphincter function. A relapsing course is common, and may continue for weeks or months.

Recurrent herpes simplex. After a primary infection, recurrent mucocutaneous lesions may occur, so-called 'cold sores'. Recurrences may be precipitated by sunburn, trauma or infections, particularly pneumococcal and meningococcal disease. Pain and redness slightly precedes the appearance of a group of small vesicles, which gradually heal in a week or two by scabbing.

Cutaneous herpes simplex. Cutaneous lesions may occur, often on the face or buttock, or in the finger pulp. Painful nodules rapidly develop to vesicles, or groups of vesicles, and in soft skin these sometimes coalesce to form bullae. Single vesicles can be difficult to distinguish clinically from the tender vesicle or pustule sometimes seen in gonococcal bacteraemia.

Dendritic ulcer. This is an irregular, branching ulcer of the cornea, which may impair vision if it is large or central. It is one cause of a painful red eye. The epithelial defect will show as yellow-green fluorescence after instillation of fluorescein drops, but may be difficult to see without expert slit-lamp examination. A red eye in a patient with a 'cold sore' is particularly likely to be caused by a dendritic ulcer.

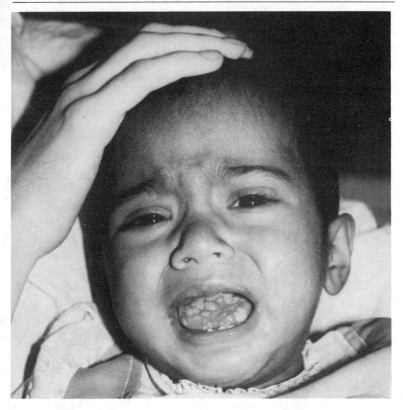

Fig. 2. Primary herpetic stomatitis.

Diagnosis
Swabs from the lesions, or vesicle fluid will readily produce a growth of herpes virus in tissue culture. Primary infections produce a significant rise of complement-fixing antibodies in paired sera.

Treatment
Local skin and mucosal infections will heal without specific treatment. Application of surgical spirit or gentian violet paint to skin or mucosa has little effect except possibly making secondary bacterial infection less likely. Idoxuridine 5% in dimethyl sulphoxide will abort skin lesions only if applied *before* vesicles appear.

Idoxuridine 0.1% eye drops are used to treat dendritic ulcer and should initially be instilled hourly. Idoxuridine 0.5%, or vidarabine 3% ointment may be applied less frequently. Expert follow-up is advisable.

Caution.   Eczematous skin is extremely susceptible to herpes simplex infection, which may spread and become confluent (Kaposi's varicelliform eruption or eczema herpeticum) (Fig. 3). Severe cases sometimes respond well to the new antiviral drugs, vidarabine or acyclovir. The full blood count and blood urea level should be reviewed frequently during antiviral therapy.

Herpes zoster

Epidemiology

This is the disease caused by reactivation of latent varicella zoster virus in the sensory ganglia of a patient who has previously had chickenpox

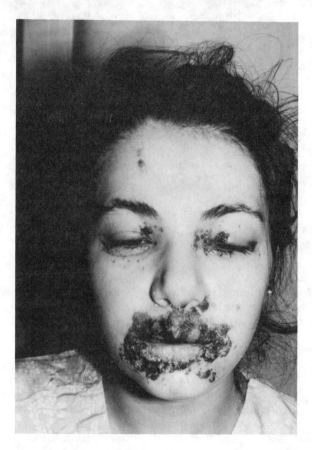

Fig. 3.   Eczema herpeticum.

(rarely it is mimicked by herpes simplex infection). Exposure to a patient with zoster is likely to result in chickenpox in susceptible individuals. The causes of virus reactivation are unknown, though trauma to the affected dermatome, feverish illness, immunosuppression and emotional shock are occasional precipitating events.

Clinical features
Pain in the affected dermatome is followed, after 1 or 2 days, by the appearance of erythema at the sites where the cutaneous nerves enter the skin. Papules, which quickly develop into clusters of coalescing vesicles, spread outwards from these sites to delineate the whole dermatome (Fig. 4a). The rash is almost always confined to one dermatome, and to one side of the body. A few chickenpox-like lesions often appear in a random distribution elsewhere, probably representing the escape of some virus from the nerves into the bloodstream.

In ophthalmic zoster, the nasociliary nerve may be involved. This results in vesicle formation on the side of the nose, and in iridocyclitis (Fig. 4b). Anterior and posterior synechiae may result if the pupil is not dilated.

The vesicles heal by crusting, a process taking from 1 week to a month or more. The lesions are infectious until they are dry.

Inflammation affects the distribution of the nerve root within the central nervous system and is associated with local meningitis. Rarely, encephalitis or lymphocytic meningitis accompanies the rash.

Caution. In patients with impaired cell-mediated immunity herpes zoster, like chickenpox, can produce a severe spreading rash and overwhelming viraemia.

Treatment
This is usually symptomatic, and includes rest and adequate analgesics. Homatropine eye drops should be administered twice daily to dilate the pupil and avoid synechiae in cases of ophthalmic zoster with iridocyclitis.

In complicated or life-threatening cases vidarabine or acyclovir may be used.

Complications
The lesions can become secondarily infected with staphylococci or streptococci. Such infections usually respond to oral flucloxacillin therapy (see impetigo). Severe disease may be complicated by septicaemia.

Severe pain (postherpetic neuralgia), sometimes persists long after the lesions, especially in the elderly. There is no effective treatment for this, but judicious use of analgesics and hypnotics may help a little.

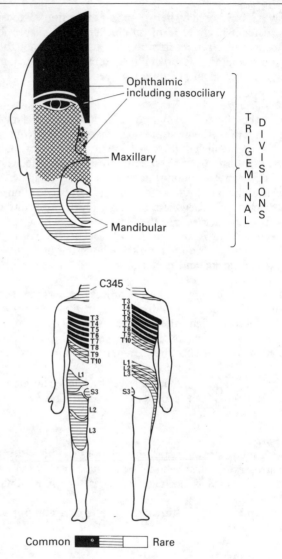

Fig. 4a   Relative frequency of segmental involvement in herpes zoster.

Cowpox and orf

These are viral infections of the hands of those who attend to cows (especially milking) and sheep (especially lambing). They are acquired by contact. Cowpox produces one or more large papules which evolve to

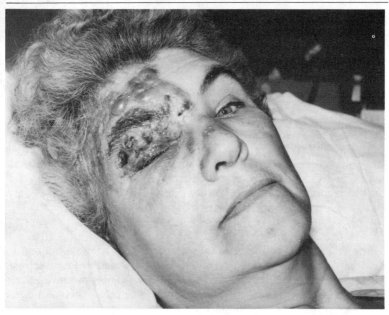

Fig. 4b. Ophthalmic herpes zoster with nasociliary involvement.

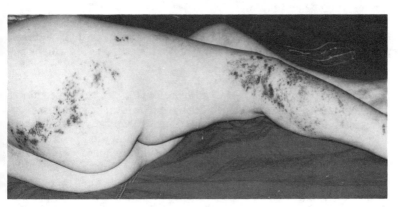

Fig. 4c. Herpes zoster of the S1 segment.

vesicles, pustules and crusts, while orf produces a large papule with a pale centre. Electron microscopy demonstrates brick-shaped pox-viruses in the vesicle fluid or tissue of the lesion. Both types of lesion heal slowly without specific therapy.

Staphylococcal skin infections

Epidemiology
Staphylococcus epidermidis (albus) and *Staph. aureus*, Gram-positive cocci, are colonists of skin, especially of the perineum, and of the external nares. *Staph. aureus* is highly pathogenic, and enters the tissues easily via small skin defects. It can be passed from person to person by contact, and can survive for some time in layers of dust. *Staph. epidermidis* is only pathogenic in a few special situations.

Clinical features
Impetigo. This is a superficial infection of the epidermis, common in children. It often begins near the nose. A brownish-yellow weeping, crusting lesion spreads slowly, and autoinoculation may produce lesions elsewhere. The condition is highly infectious. The lesions of insect bites, or chickenpox easily become impetiginized.

Occasionally *Streptococcus pyogenes* is found in impetigo lesions, which may then have a bullous element.

Boils and furunculosis. Infection of one or more hair follicles produces tender, red nodules which suppurate, and eventually break at the skin surface ('point') and drain.

Carbuncles. These are complex infections of many hair follicles, usually at the back of the neck. They are red, tender masses which contain several draining sinuses.

Pemphigus neonatorum (Lyell's syndrome). This is a rare infection of infants, in which large infected, epidermal bullae form and rupture, leaving extensive raw areas. It is caused by strains of *Staph. aureus* which produce exfoliative toxins. Without treatment the condition is often fatal. More common neonatal staphylococcal lesions include conjunctivitis and umbilical sepsis.

Toxic shock syndrome. This is a rare toxaemic illness found in patients infected with a strain of *Staph. aureus* which produces enterotoxin F. The staphylococcus is usually found in the vagina and tampon of a menstruating woman, but occasionally occurs in abscesses in others, including men and children. The illness begins with high fever and diarrhoea. After about 1 day the buccal, conjuctival and genital mucosae become reddened and a generalized macular erythema appears. This is followed by profound shock. Severe myalgia is a common feature. The plasma calcium and platelet count are low, and skeletal muscle enzymes are elevated. Blood cultures are negative. The rash and fever can be mistaken for scarlet fever or severe rubella.

Diagnosis
In all cases *Staph. aureus* can be cultured from swabs, or from pus.

Treatment
Many staphylococci are penicillinase producers, and should be treated with cloxacillin or flucloxacillin. For superficial infections oral treatment is satisfactory. This is also effective against *Streptococcus pyogenes* in impetigo lesions (important as these are sometimes nephritogenic strains). For deeper and more severe infections, intramuscular or intravenous treatment is required. Useful alternatives are cephalosporins and erythromycin.

Prevention
Washing the skin with chlorhexidine-containing agents will reduce skin carriage of staphylococci. Nasal carriage can be treated with chlorhexidine 0.1% and neomycin 0.5% cream applied twice daily for 10 days. Adequate dusting and drying of work surfaces is important in clinics and hospitals. Children with impetigo should not attend school.

Streptococcal infections

Epidemiology
Streptococcus pyogenes (Lancefield group A, beta-haemolytic streptococcus) is a Gram-positive coccus which is found on skin and in the pharynx. It enters skin defects, and passes from person to person by contact, as does *Staph. aureus*. It can also be transmitted by droplet infection and, sometimes, by food.

Clinical features
Impetigo. *Strep. pyogenes* is the cause of a minority of cases of impetigo, but should always be considered, as strains causing impetigo may precipitate nephritis (see Chapter 21).

Erysipelas. This is a superficial spreading infection in the epidermis, usually of the face or lower leg. In some cases a cut, ulcer or fissure is detectable as the site of entry of infection. The affected area of tender, red, oedematous skin is sharply demarcated from normal skin (Fig. 5). The draining lymph nodes may be enlarged. Bullae and fissures sometimes appear in the lesion. Healing is associated with desquamation.

Cellulitis. This is an infection of subcutaneous tissue in which a red,

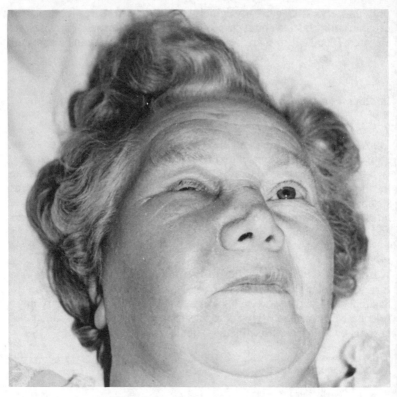

Fig. 5. Erysipelas of the face showing sharply demarcated, oedematous lesion.

tender, indurated area merges gradually into normal skin. In domiciliary practice cellulitis is often streptococcal, but it can also be staphylococcal or, in hospital practice, due to the prevalent organisms in the environment. Surgical incisions and intravenous cannulae often provide a portal of entry for such infections.

Diagnosis
The clinical picture is often sufficiently characteristic to suggest the diagnosis. Swabs from exudate, raw areas or bullae will produce a growth of beta-haemolytic streptococci in culture. Blood cultures are occasionally positive.

Serology.   If previous antibiotic treatment has made culture of the streptococci impossible, the Antistreptolysin O titre (ASOT) can be helpful. A titre of more than 250 u/ml indicates likely recent infection with *Strep. pyogenes.*

Caution. In small children cellulitis of the face or orbit is sometimes due to *Haemophilus influenzae.* This is more common on the American continent, where *H. influenzae* is relatively more prevalent than in Europe. There is a marked polymorph leukocytosis, and blood cultures are often positive.

Treatment
These are potentially serious parenchymal infections, for which the treatment of choice is parenteral benzylpenicillin. Suitable alternatives are cephaloridine, cephalothin or erythromycin. Treatment is usually continued for 7 days. Even with careful treatment erysipelas may recur, often in the same site. It can be treated with a further course of the same antibiotic as was used in the first attack.

Cutaneous diphtheria

In susceptible individuals *Corynebacterium diphtheriae* can colonize small defects in the skin. Scratches, insect bites or chickenpox lesions become inflamed, and develop a dirty whitish membrane, and serosanguineous exudate. *C. diphtheriae* can be cultured from swabs and may be toxigenic. The infection must be treated as diphtheria in all respects.

Erysipeloid

Erysipelothrix rhusiopathiae, a Gram-positive rod, is a pathogen of animals which can be acquired by those handling raw fish or meat. Usually on a finger, a sore, irritating area becomes dusky red, raised and indurated. Rarely, septicaemia or endocarditis ensue.

Culture of a small biopsy, or occasionally of a swab, will confirm the diagnosis. Oral erythromycin or intramuscular benzylpencillin provide effective treatment.

Candidiasis

Epidemiology
Candida albicans is a yeast-like fungus, which is a commensal of the skin, mouth, vagina and large bowel. Under certain conditions it becomes pathogenic and causes local disease. Predisposing factors include altered environment, such as wetness of the skin, or altered local flora after broad-spectrum antibiotic treatment. Impaired immunity due to disease or drugs, diabetes mellitus, thyrotoxicosis, hyperparathyroidism and pregnancy may be associated with candidiasis.

Clinical features
Mucosal candidiasis ('thrush').　　This can affect the mouth at any age, the

vagina of adult women and the glans penis of children or adults. It is commonly seen in diabetes mellitus, and during antibiotic therapy. The mucosa becomes red and sore with firmly attached white spots and plaques. In vaginal candidiasis there is also pruritis, oedema and a curdy discharge.

Skin candidiasis. Often seen in damp macerated skin, it produces redness and irritation in skin folds (intertrigo) or bolster-like red swelling around the nail folds (paronychia).

Diagnosis
Swabs or scrapings will readily produce a growth of *Candida albicans* on culture, and budding yeasts may be seen on microscopy of vaginal discharge.

Treatment
Many creams are available for use on the skin and vaginal mucosa. These include nystatin, miconazole, clotrimazole and econazole. Pessaries are available in doses ranging from one daily for 3 days (econazole) up to two daily for 2 weeks (nystatin).

For oral use amphotericin or nystatin suspension 1.0 ml 6-hourly, or amphotericin lozenges one or two 6-hourly, are available.

Ringworm (tinea)

Epidemiology
This is a group of fungus infections of the skin in which keratin is damaged. Species of *Trichophyton*, *Epidermophyton* and, in the scalp, *Microsporon* are responsible. Spread is by direct contact or by communal bathing and sharing of towels. Household pets may share a ringworm infection with the family.

Clinical features
Skin lesions are discoid, with a brownish, scaly, circular advancing edge. Hairs on affected skin are attacked by fungus, and break off. Typical sites are the hands or heads of children, the groin of men (*tinea cruris*) or the toe webs (*tinea pedis*). Nails are attacked by *T. rubrum*, and slowly become yellow, opaque and distorted, staring from the tip.

Diagnosis
Tinea capitis produces turquoise fluorescence under an ultraviolet (Wood's) light. Fungal mycelium is seen on microscopy of scraped-off scales, or pulled-out hairs, viewed in a few drops of 10% potassium hydroxide on a microscope slide. Hairs or scrapings can be cultured.

Caution. Erythrasma, an infection of the flexures due to *Coryne-*

bacterium minutissimum is also a cause of reddish, discoid lesions. These fluoresce coral pink under the Wood's light. Oral erythromycin is then the treatment of choice.

Treatment

Tinea pedis and tinea cruris often respond, over a few weeks, to application of clotrimazole or miconazole cream. Tinea capitis and *T. rubrum* infections are treated with oral griseofulvin. Treatment should last at least 6 weeks, and may extend over a year for nail infections.

Pityriasis versicolor

This is a common and very mild fungal infection due to *Malassezia furfur*. It produces pale fawn, irregular areas on the upper trunk. These lesions fluoresce greyish-yellow under the Wood's light. Examination of scrapings in 10% potassium hydroxide will reveal the mycelium. It may be treated with clotrimazole or miconazole cream, or with Whitfield's ointment, but usually it soon recurs.

Scabies

Epidemiology

This is an infestation with the mite *Sarcoptes scabei* which burrows under the keratinous layer of the epidermis. Young mites pass from the skin of one person to another during close prolonged contact, as in a shared bed. Transmission between sexual partners or family members is therefore common. Fertile females burrow into the skin, and lay eggs as they progress. The female dies after a few weeks, and the larvae again emerge on the skin surface.

Clinical features

Tiny, raised burrows appear in the soft skin of the axillae, wrists, elbows, finger webs, buttocks and perineum. After 3 or 4 weeks an inflammatory reaction occurs, and itchy red patches around the burrows are scratched by the patient and often become scabbed. Except in babies or in very severe attacks, the face is spared.

Diagnosis

The mite is visible as a tiny grey dot at the end of the burrow. It can be lifted out with a sharp needle, and identified by microscopy.

Treatment

All members of a household should be treated simultaneously. Traditionally two applications of benzyl benzoate paint are given on consecutive days, followed by laundry of clothes and bed linen. The whole body from the neck downwards should be treated. Unfortunately benzyl benzoate irritates the skin and can cause severe reactions in small children.

Monosulphiram lotion may be applied on two or three consecutive days or gammabenzene hexachloride cream on two consecutive days (this preparation is not irritant, and is able to kill unhatched eggs).

Caution.   If any monosulphiram is absorbed, it will have the same adverse interaction with alcohol as disulphiram (Antabuse).

Pediculosis

Gammabenzene hexachloride application, cream, lotion and shampoo are effective against most lice, but malathion preparations will cure pediculosis resistant to other therapy. Monosulphiram can also be used.

Conjunctivitis

Epidemiology
Many different organisms are firmly associated with conjunctivitis, though some, such as *Staphylococcus aureus* are cultured with equal frequency from inflamed or normal eyes. Adenoviruses are by far the commonest viral pathogens, transmitted by droplet infection and shared towels or handkerchiefs. Adenovirus type 8 can exist on tonometers and other eye instruments, and causes outbreaks of conjunctivitis in regular clinic attenders ('shipyard eye'). A recent worldwide outbreak of haemorrhagic conjunctivitis has been found to be due to enterovirus type 70. *Streptococcus pneumoniae* and *Haemophilus influenzae* are common bacterial pathogens, the latter often also causing otitis media. *Moraxella spp.* can cause outbreaks in schools and institutions, being spread by towels, handkerchiefs and makeup applicators.

Chlamydia trachomatis causes trachoma, commonly seen in crowded, rural communities in warm climates. A milder type of conjunctivitis can be caused by the types of *Chlamydia trachomatis* associated with sexually transmitted diseases.

Caution.   *Ophthalmia neonatorum*, due to either *Neisseria gonorrhoeae* or *Chlamydia trachomatis*, is severe conjunctivitis of the newborn, contracted from the mother's birth canal. In such cases, the mother *and* father, as well as the child should be offered investigation and treatment.

Clinical features
These are similar in most cases, consisting of redness and irritability of the eye, sometimes with oedema of the lids. Bacterial and neonatal infections are more likely to cause purulent exudate. In established trachoma,

follicles appear on the palpebral conjunctiva, and a layer of inflammatory tissue (pannus) may spread across the conjunctiva and cornea. Progressive fibrosis often leads to permanent blindness.

Diagnosis
Bacterial pathogens are readily isolated by culture of swabs. Adenoviruses can be isolated in tissue culture. Some centres provide diagnosis of chlamydial infection by tissue culture.

Treatment
Chloramphenicol eye drops and ointment are effective against most bacterial pathogens, and are often given in viral infections to allay secondary bacterial infection. Neomycin, framycetin and gentamicin preparations are also available, but are rarely effective against pneumococci. Sulphacetamide drops are rarely effective against *H. influenzae.*

Chlamydial infections are treated with tetracycline eye drops and ointment, usually supplemented with oral erythromycin. At least 3 weeks' treatment is recommended.

Kawasaki disease (mucocutaneous lymph node syndrome)

This is a rare disease of children, first described and more commonly seen in Japan. It consists of a feverish illness with reddening of the hands and feet, and conjunctival inflammation. The buccal mucosa becomes fissured and excoriated, and many lymph nodes are palpable. As the illness progresses, hepatic dysfunction, mucocoele of the gallbladder or aseptic meningitis may occur. Occasionally death follows, and postmortem findings suggest polyarteritis nodosa with myocardial ischaemia. Most often recovery takes up to 3 weeks, during which time a characteristic peeling of the skin and nail folds is seen.

Diagnosis is by exclusion. Bacteriological cultures and serological screening are usually negative for known pathogens. The evolution of the illness is the best clue to diagnosis. There is no known effective treatment.

Infected bites and scratches

Many animals have a varied oral flora of aerobes, anaerobes and fungi. Man has the largest repertoire of all, so that skin lesions caused by human teeth are often extensively infected, requiring a combination of benzylpenicillin and metronidazole for effective treatment.

Dog and cat bites often result in local infection caused by *Pasteurella multocida*, a Gram-negative rod which is identified by culture. Intramuscular benzylpenicillin is the best treatment. The organism is variably sensitive to other antibiotics.

Cat scratch fever may be a chlamydial infection. It follows cat scratches or bites. In 2 or 3 days an indurated swelling appears, followed after a month or so by enlargement of local lymph nodes, which may suppurate.

Antibiotics are ineffective, though aspiration of pus from the enlarged nodes may be helpful. The condition resolves in 2 to 3 months.

Drugs mentioned in this chapter

Drug	Indication	Dosage and precautions
Acyclovir	Herpes simplex	Dose for adult or child 5 mg/kg 8-hourly by slow intravenous infusion; do not give dose over less than 1 hour, or the urea will rise; check blood counts and blood urea; give 5 days' course
	Varicella zoster or very severe herpes simplex	Twice the above dose in a 5–10 days' course
Benzylpenicillin	Streptococcal skin infections	Adult dose 600 mg to 1.2 g (1–2 mega units) 6-hourly by intramuscular or intravenous injection; child's dose is a quarter to half of adult dose
Cephalexin	Mild staphylococcal or streptococcal skin infections	Adult dose 250–500 mg 6-hourly orally; child's dose is a quarter to half of adult dose
Cephaloridine	Staphylococcal or streptococcal skin infections	Adult dose 500 mg to 1.0 g 8–12 hourly by intramuscular or intravenous injection; child's dose 20–40 mg/kg daily in divided doses; can cause rising blood urea, especially if powerful diuretics are also given
Cephalothin	As above	Adult dose 1.0 g 4–6 hourly by intravenous injection; child's dose 12.5–25 mg/kg 6-hourly
Erythromycin	Streptococcal skin infections; erythrasma	Adult dose 250–500 mg 6-hourly orally or by intravenous injection or infusion; child's dose 30–35 mg/kg daily in four divided doses
Flucloxacillin Cloxacillin	Staphylococcal infections; impetigo in all cases	Adult dose 250–500 mg 6-hourly orally or by intramuscular injection. Double this dose can be given by intravenous injection or

		infusion; child's dose a quarter to half of adult dose
Griseofulvin	Fungal infections of skin and nails	Adult dose 1.0 g daily. This drug is an enzyme-inducer and reduces the efficacy of anticoagulants and oral contraceptives; child's dose 10 mg/kg daily (can be divided); continue for 4 weeks after clinical healing
Vidarabine	Herpes simplex and varicella zoster infection	Dose for adult or child 10 mg/kg daily by slow intravenous injection; continue for 5 days; check blood count

3

Mouth and Throat Infections

Introduction
The tissues of the throat are the meeting place of buccal and respiratory mucosae, and of lymphatic tissue, and this situation predisposes the area to a wide variety of infections. Many systemic diseases including chicken-pox, measles, mumps, polio, tuberculosis and syphilis can affect the mouth and throat, and should be considered, however briefly, in a differential diagnosis.

Caution. Non-infectious conditions affecting the region are also numerous; allergic reactions, drug reactions, reticuloses and leukaemia frequently cause sore throat, and result in diagnostic confusion.

Diagnostic methods
Microscopy. Light microscopy is of limited value, as the normal flora of the region includes Gram-positive cocci and Gram-negative rods identical to the expected pathogens. The spirochaetal and fusiform organisms associated with Vincent's angina, and the treponeme of syphilis can be identified, however.

Culture. Most bacterial pathogens are easily cultured from swabs. Enteroviruses, adenoviruses and the viruses of influenza can be isolated in tissue culture. Enteroviruses and adenoviruses can also be recovered from stool cultures, for they usually colonize the bowel in large numbers.

Serology. Complement-fixing antibodies to many viral pathogens can be detected in patients' serum. The antistreptolysin O titre (ASOT) is useful in making a retrospective diagnosis of *Streptococcus pyogenes* infection.

Viral pharyngitis

Epidemiology
Most of the many respiratory pathogens can cause pharyngitis. These include agents of the common cold, and ECHO, coxsackie, polio, adenoviruses, influenza viruses, measles and rubella. Most spread by

droplet transmission, but the first three (the enteroviruses) and adenoviruses are excreted in the stool and can also be spread by the faecal–oral route. The prevalence of particular viral pathogens varies throughout the year, each virus having a characteristic time of peak incidence.

Clinical features
Most viral throat infections consist of a brief feverish illness with a varying degree of redness of the fauces and soft palate. The tonsils may also be enlarged. Pain is not well related to the degree of visible inflammation. Generalized myalgia is a common complaint and the patient may notice moderate enlargement of lymph nodes in the cervical region.

Rashes. Coxsackie group A infections can produce an enanthem of shallow, red-rimmed ulcers on the palate and fauces. Indeed coxsackie A-16 may also cause a rash of small, superficial blisters on the hands and feet, often with a papulovesicular eruption on the buttocks. This disorder, called hand, foot and mouth disease, is highly infectious and is common in toddlers.

All of the viruses, particularly ECHO and coxsackie will sometimes produce a generalized maculopapular rash. On rare occasions coxsackie infections are associated with a vesicular eruption.

Other associated features. Severe myalgia mimicking pleurisy or peritonitis can occur in coxsackie group B infections. This is called Bornholm disease or epidemic myalgia, and is usually associated with high fever and severe pharyngitis.

Conjunctivitis, due to adenovirus infection, may be associated with pharyngitis and painful enlargement of cervical lymph nodes. This condition is called pharyngoconjunctival fever.

Orchitis and myocarditis are occasional accompaniments of coxsackie infections. Pericarditis can follow mild pharyngitis due to a variety of viral agents.

Diagnosis
The cervical lymphadenopathy, normal white blood cell count and associated myalgia will suggest a viral aetiology. Tissue culture of material from throat swabs or stools may produce an identifiable viral agent. Complement fixation tests for viral antibodies can be used to screen acute and convalescent sera for significant rising titres, but are not always reliable particularly in coxsackie infections.

Treatment
No specific antiviral therapy is yet available for the treatment of pharyngitis. The value of bedrest in shortening the illness and relieving distress should not be underestimated. Aspirin and other non-steroidal

anti-inflammatory agents (NSAID) can greatly reduce pain and swelling. A useful regimen is 600 mg soluble aspirin in a tumbler of water, to be gargled and swallowed 6-hourly (50 mg/kg daily in divided doses for children over age 1).

Infectious mononucleosis

Epidemiology
Epstein–Barr virus is a herpes-like virus which is widespread in the population. It is probably spread by droplet transmission, requiring close contact for infection to take place. Infectious mononucleosis is a result of primary E–B virus infection, and mainly affects those in the teens and twenties, though no age-group is exempt. Reactivation of E–B virus in the tissues may play a part in the occurrence of certain reticuloses, such as Burkitt's lymphoma.

Clinical features
There are three main clinical types of infectious mononucleosis.

Anginose form.   This is the typical 'glandular fever' syndrome, with sore throat and widespread lymphadenopathy. The fauces and palate become extremely oedematous, as often do the tissues of the eyelids, nasal passages and neck. The tonsils become partly or completely covered with a foamy cream or white exudate (Fig. 6a) which hardly ever extends to mucosal surfaces. A rash of petechiae often appears at the junction of the hard and soft palate. Severe pharyngeal oedema can cause respiratory obstruction. Warning signs are rapid pulse, noisy breathing and inability to swallow saliva.

Enlarged lymph nodes can be found in many regions, sometimes including the epitrochlear and occipital sites. In up to half of patients the spleen becomes palpable.

A small percentage of patients develop a fine maculopapular rash on the extensor surfaces. This rarely appears before the second week.

Hepatitic form.   Elevation of aspartate transaminase levels is usual in infectious mononucleosis, but clinical jaundice is uncommon. Occasionally, however, a case presents as 'infectious hepatitis'. Fever is usually marked, but lymph node enlargment may be minimal. Even in the absence of sore throat, petechiae or exudate are sometimes seen in the mouth.

Febrile form.   This presents simply as a feverish illness, sometimes with lymph node enlargement and signs in the mouth. Left hypochondrial pain due to 'perisplenitis' may suggest the correct diagnosis. Small children commonly suffer from this type of infection.

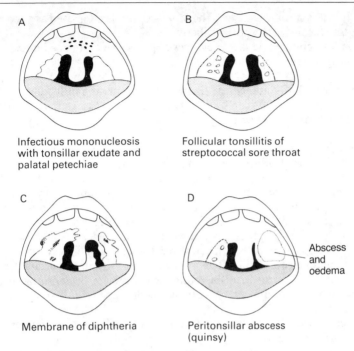

A. Infectious mononucleosis with tonsillar exudate and palatal petechiae

B. Follicular tonsillitis of streptococcal sore throat

C. Membrane of diphtheria

D. Peritonsillar abscess (quinsy) — Abscess and oedema

Fig. 6. Appearances of the throat in different infections.

Other features. Electrocardiographic abnormalities are common; occasionally clinically evident myocarditis occurs. Proteinuria may be seen, but rarely indicates severe nephritis. Other occasional findings are meningoencephalitis, cranial and peripheral nerve lesions, autoimmune haemolytic anaemia and thrombocytopenia.

Diagnosis
Clinical features may be diagnostic, but are not always easy to distinguish from streptococcal follicular tonsillitis, or from diphtheria. In the blood film up to 50% of lymphocytes are atypical, appearing larger than usual with evidence of extreme metabolic activity.

The Paul–Bunnell test. An antibody which agglutinates sheep red blood cells (a heterophil antibody) appears in the serum of cases after the first to third week, and may persist for several months. It can be confirmed as the true Paul–Bunnell antibody by absorption of the serum with guineapig kidney cells (which removes most non-specific heterophil antibodies) and with ox red blood cells (which removes the Paul–Bunnell antibody). A slightly less specific slide test, the *Monospot test* is often used as a screening test for the heterophil antibody.

Small children may not develop positive Paul–Bunnell or Monospot tests.

Serology.   Both complement-fixing and agglutinating antibodies to viral capsid antigen (VCA) can be detected in IgG or IgM fractions, if retrospective diagnosis is necessary.

Other causes of glandular fever syndromes.   Toxoplasmosis commonly causes a feverish illness with lymph node enlargement. If affects particularly those in their teens and twenties. The lymphadenopathy is often confined to one region or group of nodes and is accompanied by an atypical lymphocytosis but rarely of the degree seen in infectious mononucleosis. The diagnosis is serological, based on the toxoplasma dye test or the haemagglutination test, in single or paired sera.

Cytomegalovirus infection can also cause a feverish illness with atypical mononucleosis, and often with elevation of the aspartate transaminase. The virus can be cultivated from early morning urine specimens, and complement-fixing antibodies appear in rising titres in the serum.

Neither toxoplasmosis nor cytomegalovirus infection cause a positive Paul–Bunnell test.

Treatment
This is the same as for other viral pharyngeal infections. Antibiotics are not indicated, indeed the majority of patients with infectious mononucleosis will develop an itching maculopapular rash if treated with ampicillin or related drugs.

Respiratory obstruction.   Threatened obstruction may be averted by giving 200 mg hydrocortisone intravenously as a bolus. This reduces oedema, but does not affect the course of the disease. Several doses may be needed to maintain improvement, and aspirin gargles may contribute an anti-inflammatory effect. In extreme cases tracheostomy is indicated.

Autoimmune manifestations.   Anaemia or thrombocytopenia is occasionally severe. High doses of prednisolone will often ameliorate the problem, which rarely lasts more than 2 or 3 weeks.

Splenic rupture.   This is a rare but life-threatening event. Repeated palpation of the enlarged spleen should be avoided, and severe abdominal pain should be regarded seriously.

Postviral aesthenia.   Severe lassitude may persist for several weeks after resolution of the other symptoms. There is no specific treatment and sudden recovery is the usual outcome.

Streptococcal tonsillitis

Epidemiology
Streptococcus pyogenes, a beta-haemolytic, Lancefield group A streptococcus, is a Gram-positive coccus which is a common inhabitant of the skin, pharynx and nares of man. It passes by contact or droplet transmission from person to person, and some of those who acquire it will become ill. Outbreaks of streptococcal tonsillitis are common in boarding schools and residential institutions.

The importance of outbreaks rests not only in the potential severity of the illness, but in the likelihood of associated poststreptococcal states, particularly nephritis and rheumatic fever (see Chapter 21).

Clinical features
Fever, chills and sore throat develop quickly after the incubation period of 2 or 3 days. In contrast to patients with viral infections, who feel uncomfortable and tired, those with streptococcal infections often feel very ill.

The palate and fauces are red, and the tonsils are enlarged, with dots of white exudate arising from the crypts (Fig. 6b). The draining lymph nodes at the angles of the jaw become enlarged and tender.

There is a neutrophil leukocytosis, usually with a white cell count of $11–15 \times 10^9$/l of which 80% or more are neutrophils. Children under age 2 may not have such a high white cell count, as their neutrophil response is not well developed.

Quinsy. This is a peritonsillar abscess. A boggy oedematous swelling involves the palate and fauces surrounding the affected tonsil. It hangs from one side of the palate, and presses sideways against the upper molars (Fig. 6d). Pus may point and drain into the pharynx. Bilateral quinsies can produce enough swelling to cause significant respiratory obstruction.

Scarlet fever. This is a toxic illness with a rash. It occurs when the infecting *Strep. pyogenes* produces an erythrogenic toxin. Although it usually accompanies sore throat, scarlet fever may originate from infection of skin lesions, when it is called surgical scarlet fever. The rash (a punctate erythema) is formed by the merging of many small macules, with exaggerated, easily palpable hair follicles. The rash is exaggerated in the skin folds (Pastia's sign). The skin looks and feels like red sandpaper, but the perioral skin is often spared. The tongue is furred, with red papillae (white strawberry tongue), and peels from the tip in 2 or 3 days to become red (red strawberry tongue).

Caution.   The rash of scarlet fever is similar to that of toxic shock syndrome and of severe rubella. The three diseases can be difficult to distinguish in their early stages if an associated tonsillitis, abscess or vaginal infection is not obvious.

Diagnosis
Throat swabs will produce a growth of beta-haemolytic streptococci in culture. However, such streptococci are not always pathogenic, for instance they are sometimes recovered from the throats of asymptomatic carriers or patients with infectious mononucleosis. Clinical judgement must therefore be applied to decide the importance of cultural findings.

Serology   The serum antistreptolysin-O titre (ASOT) is useful in making a retrospective diagnosis, or when antibiotic treatment has made culture impossible. It also helps to distinguish infected individuals from passive carriers. A titre of more than 250 u/ml indicates recent infection. Paired sera may reveal a significant rise in ASOT.

Other antistreptococcal antibodies estimated for epidemiological purposes include antiDNAase B and antihyaluronidase.

Treatment
The treatment of choice is intramuscular benzylpenicillin. Suitable alternatives are erythromycin or narrow spectrum cephalosporins such as cephalothin. Treatment is usually continued for 10 days. Oral medication may replace parenteral treatment when the temperature has returned to normal.

Scarlet fever.   Will respond to the same treatment as streptococcal sore throat.

Quinsy.   This will often resolve or drain spontaneously during penicillin treatment, though high doses are required to penetrate the oedematous tissue. A persistent abscess or bilateral abscesses threatening the airway may require incision. This is best carried out by an experienced operator, as palatal arteries and nerves pass through the area of the abscess.

Caution.   Carriers of *Strep. pyogenes* in a closed community may be a source of repeated epidemics. Oral penicillin therapy rarely eradicates the carrier state, indeed a 7–10 days course of intramuscular penicillin may be required. Neomycin and chlorhexidine cream is helpful in eradicating nasal organisms.

Acute epiglottitis

Epidemiology
This is a severe, life-threatening infection caused by *Haemophilus influenzae*, a Gram-negative rod which exists in the nasopharynx. It

spreads by droplet infection, and is particularly likely to cause disease in children below age 5, though older children and adults are sometimes affected.

Clinical features
Typically these consist of feverish illness with rapidly worsening sore throat, dysphagia and eventually, respiratory obstruction. Inability to swallow saliva is a sinister sign.

If the tongue is depressed with a spatula, the bright red, oedematous, cherry-like epiglottis is seen at its base. There is a risk that examination may finally precipitate obstruction if the airway is threatened.

Diagnosis
The clinical features are usually sufficient grounds for diagnosis. If emergency X-ray facilities are available, a lateral view of the soft tissues of the neck will reveal the spherical mass of the swollen epiglottis (Fig. 7) and obviate the risk of clinical examination, but the greatest risk is of delay in diagnosis.

There is a high neutrophil leukocytosis; throat swabs and blood cultures often produce a growth of *H. influenzae*.

Treatment
Facilities for tracheostomy should be available. Local oedema may be reduced by intravenous hydrocortisone 200 mg.

The antibiotic of choice is chloramphenicol, which should be given intravenously as soon as culture specimens have been obtained. Chloramphenicol may be given orally as soon as the patient can swallow it, as absorption from the gut is excellent. Treatment is continued for 7–10 days.

Ampicillin is a suitable alternative for sensitive *H.influenzae*, but there is an increasing risk that the organism will be ampicillin-resistant.

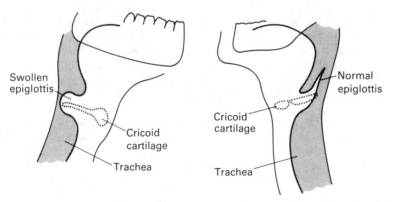

Fig. 7. Appearance of lateral X-ray of the soft tissues of the neck in acute epiglottitis.

Diphtheria

Epidemiology

This is a disease due to *Corynebacterium diphtheriae*, a Gram-positive rod which produces a potent exotoxin. Three main strains exist: gravis, intermedius and mitis, in toxigenic and non-toxigenic variants. *C. ulcerans*, a pathogen predominantly of cows, also produces toxin and can infect humans. Unimmunized individuals and communities throughout the world are susceptible to diphtheria, and infection is acquired by close contact with cases or carriers. Children are more often affected than adults as immunity often develops with age.

Clinical features

The usual incubation period is 1–3 days. The most common site affected is the pharynx, which becomes inflamed and develops a greyish *membrane*, a tough exudate of fibrin and dead cells which adheres firmly to the mucosa, and often becomes discoloured or bloodstained. The disease may affect the tonsils, pharynx, nares, conjunctiva or trachea, larynx and bronchial tree. In contrast with the exudate of infectious mononucleosis, the membrane of diphtheria is not confined to the tonsils (Fig. 6c). Nasal, conjunctival or laryngeal diphtheria without tonsillar exudate is a recognized diagnostic pitfall. Croup is a common feature of tracheal and laryngeal disease.

Occasionally scratches, insect bites or chickenpox lesions become infected and develop a membrane with a serosanguineous exudate. This situation can be dangerous because, as in mucosal infections toxin can be produced in the lesions.

Although the temperature is rarely very high, there may be intense swelling of the tissues of the neck (bull neck) and of the tonsillar lymph nodes. The patient is listless and ill due to the effects of the toxin, and tachycardia is often out of proportion to the slight fever.

Myocardial damage. Myocarditis becomes evident during the second week of illness, and is due to destruction of myocardial cells by toxin. A variety of electrocardiographic abnormalities may occur, including abnormal P- and T- waves, extrasystoles, tachycardias and heart block. Clinically obvious heart failure may develop, and is difficult to treat as digoxin may exacerbate heart block and is therefore contraindicated. If the patient recovers, myocardial recovery is complete in a few weeks.

Nervous system damage. This is due to demyelination of motor nerves, and occurs from the third week of illness. The most common lesions are paralysis of the palate, or of extraocular muscles. Less frequently pharyngeal or laryngeal paralysis occur, and paralysis of limbs or of respiratory muscles is rare.

Renal and adrenal damage. Although transient proteinuria is commonly seen, severe renal failure is rare. Adrenal failure usually accompanies renal failure.

Diagnosis

All unimmunized individuals are likely to be susceptible. Even in western countries there are groups and communities who refuse or neglect childhood immunization, so that the physician must always consider diphtheria in the differential diagnosis of sore throat, exudative pharyngitis, croup or stridor.

A slight neutrophil leukocytosis is usually present. Nose or throat swabs produce a growth of *C. diphtheriae* except after recent antibiotic treatment.

The Schick test. This intradermal test will detect susceptible individuals in 1–2 days. Toxin 0.2 ml is given in the left forearm, and inactivated toxin in the right. The appearance of a red reaction on the left arm indicates susceptibility. In some cases the right arm reddens equally, demonstrating hypersensitivity to an antigen other than the toxin. This 'false positive' response usually indicates immunity.

Treatment

The airway. Respiratory obstruction can develop rapidly. Pharyngeal and laryngeal obstruction can be bypassed by tracheostomy, but bronchial membrane may also be present. Facilities for emergency tracheostomy should be available.

Antitoxin. This is given to prevent further fixation of toxin in the tissues. It is derived from horse serum, so that a test dose of 0.1 ml is recommended to detect a possible anaphylactic reaction. If a reaction occurs intravenous hydrocortisone 200 mg and promethazine 10 mg should be given before testing further small doses.

The usual dose is 30 000–60 000 units (10 000 units for nasal or conjunctival disease, or up to 120 000 units for severe tracheobronchial disease). Up to half of the dose may be given intravenously, if there is no reaction 30 minutes after initial intramuscular dosage.

Antitoxin may be given from 6 hours after Schick testing, without affecting the result of the test.

Antibiotics. The treatment of choice is benzylpenicillin. Erythromycin is a satisfactory alternative. Dosage is continued for 10–14 days.

The carrier state. This may persist for weeks, even after penicillin treatment. Oral erythromycin will usually eradicate the organism but three or more negative nose and throat swabs should be obtained to confirm clearance, as relapse is common and a further course may be necessary.

Prevention

As with streptococcal infection, asymptomatic carriers may be the source of an outbreak. Close contacts, family, class and dormitory contacts should have nose and throat swabs. Sufferers and carriers should be isolated and treated. Any contact who develops fever or sore throat should be isolated for investigation.

Childhood immunization is safe and effective (see Chapter 20).

Vincent's angina

This is a fairly common condition due to synergistic infection with an anaerobic fusiform bacillus, and the spirochaete *Borellia vincentii*. The buccal mucosa is very red and sore, and may become shaggy and ulcerated. The gingival mucosa is often involved. An unpleasant, acidic fetor may be present.

The characteristic organisms can be seen on a Gram-stained smear of mouth swabbings.

Eradication either of the fusiform bacillus with oral metronidazole, or of the spirochaete with intramuscular benzylpenicillin is effective treatment.

Ludwig's angina

This is a serious pyogenic infection of sublingual tissue planes with organisms derived from the mouth. It sometimes follows dental procedures, but often even minor trauma cannot be remembered by the patient.

The patient is feverish and ill with gross tender swelling of the neck and chin. The tissues are indurated and the overlying skin may be red. The tongue is pushed up by swelling of the floor of the mouth, which may bulge over the lower teeth. There is significant danger of respiratory obstruction.

Treatment should be begun promptly. Benzylpencillin and metronidazole are usually given together, as they are active against aerobic and anaerobic organisms. Intravenous hydrocortisone 200 mg may help to reduce the severe oedema.

If prompt improvement does not occur, the patient should be referred to an ear, nose and throat specialist for early surgical drainage of the tissue planes.

Actinomycosis

This is an unusual condition due to Gram-positive, branching organisms, *Actinomyces spp.*, which are usually found in tonsillar crypts, large bowel and other anaerobic situations.

Indolent, indurated inflammatory lesions with many draining sinuses appear in the tissues of the jaw or lower abdominal wall. They can often be related to an episode of trauma or surgery. Occasionally lesions occur on the chest wall, or in the lungs.

The pus from the sinuses contains tiny yellow dots, known as 'sulphur granules', and Gram-staining of granules will clearly show the branching structure of the organism.

Laboratory testing will reveal unpredictable sensitivity to a variety of antibiotics, but the favoured treatment is intravenous benzylpenicillin in large doses. This must often be continued for several weeks.

Acute otitis media

This is the condition of suppurative bacterial infection of the middle ear. The middle ear is an extension of the pharyngeal mucosa, and becomes stagnant and infected when the connecting Eustachian tube is blocked. Catarrhal illnesses, especially in children, precipitate fever, pain in the ear and a dusky red, bulging eardrum which may rupture and discharge pus.

The pathogens are organisms from the throat, often *Haemophilus influenzae* or *Streptococcus pneumoniae*, and are usually eradicated apparently successfully in domiciliary practice by oral ampicillin, amoxycillin or co-trimoxazole. In hospital practice intramuscular ampicillin or penicillin is usually given, depending on the organism thought to be responsible.

Chronic infections

In chronic or recurrent otitis media other organisms may become predominant. *Staphylococcus aureus* or Gram-negative rods may appear. On rare occasions *Clostridium tetani* invades a stagnant infected ear.

Drugs mentioned in this chapter

Drug	Indication	Usage and precautions
Benzylpenicillin	Drug of choice for streptococcal tonsillitis and acute diphtheria	Adult dose 600 mg to 1.2 g (1–2 mega units) 6-hourly by intramuscular or intravenous injection or infusion; dose may be doubled in peritonsillar abscess or diphtheria; child's dose is a quarter to half of adult dose
Cephalothin	Alternative to penicillin	Adult dose 1.0 g 4-hourly by intravenous injection; child's dose 12.5–25 mg/kg 6-hourly
Cephradine	Alternative to penicillin	Adult dose 500 mg–1.0 g 6-hourly by intramuscular or intravenous injection; child's dose 50–100 mg/kg daily in four divided doses

	Streptococcal carriers	Oral dose is half of intravenous dose; continue for 10–14 days
Chloramphenicol	*Haemophilus influenzae* epiglottitis	Adult dose 500 mg 6-hourly orally or intravenously (3.0 g daily may be given to large adult); child's dose 50–100 mg/kg daily in four divided doses; check the white blood cell and platelet counts
Chlorhexidine and neomycin cream	Nasal carriers of *Staphylococcus aureus*	Apply to interior of nostrils twice daily for 10 days
Diphtheria antitoxin	Acute diphtheria	This is a refined product of horse serum; obtainable from Regional Pharmacies in the UK; adult dose is 10 000–100 000 units depending on the extent of the membrane; half of the dose may be given by intravenous injection if there is no adverse reaction to intramuscular injection; child's dose is a quarter to half of adult dose
	Prophylaxis in unimmunized diphtheria carriers	Adult dose 5000 units by intramuscular injection; child's dose is a quarter to half of adult dose
Erythromycin	Alternative to penicillin for acute infections	Adult dose 300–500 mg 6-hourly by intravenous injection; child's dose 30–50 mg/kg daily in four divided doses
	Drug of choice for diphtheria carriers	Adult dose 250–500 mg 6-hourly orally; child's dose is half of adult dose
Metronidazole	Vincent's angina or acute gingivitis	Adult dose 200 mg 8-hourly orally; this drug has an 'antabuse effect' if taken with alcohol; child's dose 7.5 mg/kg 8-hourly

4

Respiratory Infections

Most respiratory pathogens are able to cause disease of both the upper and lower respiratory tract. Respiratory infections therefore usually consist of a variable combination of pharyngitis, laryngitis, tracheitis, bronchitis, bronchiolitis and pneumonia (alveolitis). Lung infection can follow invasion by flora from the upper respiratory tract, or be part of a bacteraemia or viraemia.

Symptoms and signs of respiratory infections
Cough. This is usual, and its nature may be diagnostically characteristic, as in the bovine cough of croup, or the paroxysms of pertussis. Attention should be paid to the presence and nature of sputum, for mucoid sputum usually indicates viral infection, while purulent sputum often contains bacterial pathogens. Production of several hundred millilitres of sputum daily is a sign of bronchiectasis.

Treatment of cough. Two main types of cough are distinguishable, the unproductive and the productive. An unproductive cough is often caused by mucosal irritation due to inflammation, oedema or adherent mucus or slough. This type of cough is often painful and it may increase local mucosal damage. It may also prevent adequate rest and sleep. Significant relief can be obtained simply by drinking warm fluids or by taking simple linctus. If this is not sufficient, antitussives may be used. The phenothiazines such as promethazine and trimeprazine have a mildly sedative effect, which may aid sleep. Stronger agents are codeine or pholcodine. All are available as syrup or linctus.

It may be unwise to suppress a productive cough, as this can impair clearance of infected material or obstructing mucus. Antitussives or sedatives should be used with caution in these circumstances. Expectoration is aided by good hydration, warm drinks and steam inhalations, all of which tend to liquefy mucus and mucopus. It is not essential to add aromatic tinctures to steam inhalations.

There are numerous proprietary medicines containing phenothiazine or narcotic antussive agents alone or in combination with 'expectorants' such as iodide compounds or menthol. Many of these are quite strongly sedative.

Noisy breathing.   The hollow, hissing sound of stridor emanates from a narrowed glottis, while a wheeze usually indicates bronchial or bronchiolar constriction. Obstruction of airways, in adults as well as children, will result in flaring of the ala nasae, followed by recession of intercostal tissue during inspiration. Supraclavicular and subcostal recession are seen in severe cases.

Treatment of respiratory obstruction.   Some types of respiratory obstruction are due to bronchial muscle spasm. This is common in patients who suffer from asthma or chronic bronchitis. These patients often have a history of previous attacks of wheezing, and will respond to treatment with bronchodilators such as salbutamol, terbutaline or aminophylline. In cases of croup, tracheitis and bronchitis, however, obstruction is usually due to oedema of the mucosa and adherence of tenacious mucus. In these cases humidification of the inspired air is often extremely beneficial, as it liquefies the mucus, and allows expectoration. This in turn reduces the irritation and oedema of the mucosa. Steam is the best agent, as it is a vapour and will penetrate smaller airways than droplets from a nebulizer. In the home, a hot bath may be run, or a kettle boiled in a closed room to provide a humid atmosphere; in hospital a steam kettle is used.

If respiratory obstruction threatens, rapid respiration will be accompanied by a rising pulse. Cyanosis first appears in the hands and feet and is quickly followed by central cyanosis and apnoeic attacks, which give warning of impending respiratory arrest. In these circumstances mucosal oedema can be reduced non-specifically by giving a large, intravenous dose of hydrocortisone. In croup and bronchiolitis this may avoid the need for tracheostomy or tracheal intubation. It can be repeated once or twice over a period of 12 hours.

Oxygen/humidity tents are available which will enclose a small child in a cot. Increased oxygen levels, and water from a nebulizer can be provided in such tents.

It is worth remembering that helium–oxygen (80% : 20%) mixture is available in some ear, nose and throat departments, and because of its very low viscosity it will pass effectively through airways which are too narrowed to admit sufficient air or oxygen.

Chest examination

Altered chest movement, percussion note and vocal fremitus or resonance are helpful signs in established consolidation. In the early stages, however, the only sign may be a localized patch of coarse crepitations at the end of inspiration. It is therefore important in auscultation to listen throughout the respiratory cycle in several areas, so as not to miss this finding.

The chest X-ray.   This will demonstrate an area of consolidation or a pleural effusion. It will not demonstrate dry pleurisy or pericarditis, which are detectable by hearing a pleural or pericardial rub on auscultation. It is often normal, or nearly so, in bronchitis, unless pneumonia coexists. Grossly abnormal bronchi however, as in bronchiectasis, will produce saccular, fusiform or 'tramline' opacities in the affected lung field.

Other diagnostic methods
Sputum culture.   This is commonly carried out, but is sometimes confusing, due to contamination by upper respiratory tract flora. Aspiration from the trachea by intubation or cricothyroid membrane puncture is sometimes employed to avoid this.

Percutaneous needle aspiration.   This may be carried out from *consolidated* lung. Lung biopsy is occasionally employed in special centres.

Counter immunoelectrophoresis (CIE).   This is an immunological method by which certain antigens can be detected in sputum (or serum if the antigen has entered the blood). Antigens of *Streptococcus pneumoniae* and *Haemophilus influenzae* can be detected by this means.

Caution.   The differential diagnosis of fever with abnormal findings on chest examination includes malignant infiltration, collagen diseases (especially sarcoidosis, lupus erythematosus, polyarteritis nodosa and Wegener's granulomatosis) and allergic alveolitis or pulmonary eosinophilia. Sputum cytology, blood examination for abnormal antibodies, skin tests and lung biopsy may be indicated in these cases.

Croup

Epidemiology
This is a characteristic illness predominantly of infants and children. It is a type of laryngotracheitis due to such pathogens as respiratory syncytial virus, measles virus, influenza and *Mycoplasma pneumoniae*. Outbreaks occur with epidemics of these viruses.

Caution.   Laryngeal diphtheria is a recognized cause of croup. The membrane is not always visible on pharyngeal inspection.

Clinical features
These are diagnostic. Superimposed on the features of respiratory infection (coryza, signs in the chest, etc) is the typical hollow sound of the breathing, as though through a tube, and dry, low-pitched monotonous 'bovine' cough. Accumulation of oedema and secretions can lead to respiratory obstruction, heralded by a rising pulse, and difficulty in swallowing saliva.

Diagnosis

This is clinical. The responsible pathogen may be revealed by sputum culture or by rising antibody titres in paired sera. If there is a leukocytosis, bacterial causes should be considered.

Treatment

Humidification of inspired air is most important, and in many cases this alone will be sufficient treatment to bring about a steady improvement.

If respiratory obstruction threatens, intravenous hydrocortisone will often reduce oedema. Otherwise, humidified oxygen in a cot-sized oxygen tent may be required. Tracheostomy is indicated if the airway is still inadequate.

Specific antimicrobial therapy is not usually indicated, as croup is generally due to a virus infection.

Bronchiolitis

Epidemiology

This is a disease affecting mainly infants below age 2, whose small airways easily become obstructed by oedema and thick mucus. It is usually due to respiratory syncytical virus (RSV) infection, which spreads by droplet transmission. Epidemics tend to occur in late winter.

Clinical features

At first the child appears to have a cold but after a few days persistent cough, tachycardia, intercostal recession, prolonged expiration and wheezing rapidly appear. The sputum is gelatinous or mucoid. There may be a few crepitations audible on auscultation of the chest, but the main findings are reduced air entry and expiratory wheeze. Chest X-ray shows a variable degree of emphysema and patchy atelectasis caused by partial and complete airways obstruction. Cyanosis, apnoea and death can occur suddenly in severe cases.

Diagnosis

This is clinical. Tissue culture of sputum will produce RSV or rarely another pathogen, and paired sera will demonstrate a rising titre of antibody.

Treatment

As for croup, humidity and regular removal of secretions from the throat are essential. An oxygen tent may be needed to provide a high concentration of humidified oxygen. In severe cases tracheostomy will allow the utilization of raised end-expiratory pressure to aid oxygen absorption. Intravenous hydrocortisone will sometimes ameliorate severe endo-bronchiolar oedema. Severe congestive cardiac failure may require treatment with digoxin.

After 4 or 5 days the child usually begins to improve slowly. Secondary bacterial infection is unusual.

Bronchitis and secondary chest infections

Epidemiology
Any lower respiratory tract whose natural defences have been compromised by pre-existing disease will be unusually susceptible to infection. Recognized predispositions include chronic bronchitis, mucoviscidosis, dust diseases, and recent infection with some viruses such as influenza or measles. Infection is usually due to invasion by local flora such as pneumococci (*Streptococcus pneumoniae*) or *Haemophilus influenzae*. After viral infection or antibiotic administration *Staphylococcus aureus* is a common pathogen.

Clinical features
Increasing cough and shortness of breath are accompanied by a change in the sputum from mucoid to purulent. The degree of fever is variable. Widespread increase in crepitations and rhonchi on auscultation is accompanied by a general loss of lucency of the lungs on X-ray. A localized area of consolidation may be detectable clinically and radiologically.

Diagnosis
Culture of the sputum will sometimes identify the responsible pathogen, but may simply produce a mixed growth of local flora.

Treatment
A short course of antibiotic therapy (5–7 days) is given in conjunction with vigorous general measures such as physiotherapy, bronchodilator drugs and steam inhalations. The aim is to eradicate existing infection before a more resistant local flora becomes established. Oral dosage is adequate unless infection is severe, or pneumonia coexists. Suitable drugs are ampicillin, amoxycillin or tetracycline. If *Staph. aureus* is a likely pathogen, cloxacillin or flucloxacillin should be added, or co-trimoxazole given instead. Only the widest spectrum cephalosporins are active against *H. influenzae*. Aminoglycosides are ineffective against pneumococci.

Prophylaxis. In exceptional circumstances, regular low-dose antibiotic therapy is given to alleviate incessant attacks of bronchitis. Doxycycline is often used, or in children with mucoviscidosis co-trimoxazole can be helpful.

Pneumococcal pneumonia

Epidemiology

This is the classical lobar pneumonia caused by *Streptococcus pneumoniae* and tends mainly to affect the young and middle-aged. Although droplet transmission is possible, it is likely that a change in host susceptibility is at least as important as the acquisition of the organism in the pathogenesis of this infection. Since 46 pneumococcal types, or groups of types, can be distinguished by their capsular antigens, repeated infection with different types is possible. Patients with altered immunity, hyposplenism or hepatic cirrhosis are particularly susceptible.

Clinical features

Illness begins with a high fever and non-specific symptoms such as nausea, loose stools or headache. Some patients have pleuritic pain in the affected area, often with a pleural rub, and a minority have rigors. Sweating is often surprisingly absent. After some hours or days a dry cough begins. Only at this stage do signs of consolidation appear in the chest: first, localized crepitation and soon dullness to percussion, increased vocal resonance and bronchial breathing. Rusty sputum appears as the dense consolidation begins to break down.

The blood shows a marked neutrophil leukocytosis of $18 \times 10^9/l$ or more, and chest X-ray shows a shadow delineated by the borders of a lung lobe (Fig. 8). Occasionally more than one lobe is involved. A few patients have positive blood cultures.

Diagnosis

The clinical and radiological features are often sufficient for a fairly cer-

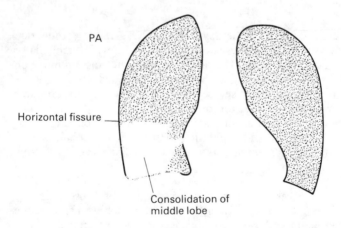

Fig: 8.   Consolidation of the middle lobe in lobar pneumonia.

tain diagnosis. As sputum appears late in the illness, it is seldom available for culture, and blood culture is often negative.

Serological tests.   Counter immunoelectrophoresis (CIE) can detect pneumococcal antigens in sputum (or in blood if there has been bacteraemia), and is a useful investigation when antibiotic treatment has made culture impossible. A rising titre of antibodies to the infecting strain will appear in the blood, but this is now rarely used as a diagnostic test.

Caution.   Occasionally young Asians present with upper lobe pneumonia, but with little change in the white cell count. Tuberculosis should be considered in the differential diagnosis of these cases.

Treatment
Oral antibiotics are rarely effective and may not prevent the development of complications. The treatment of choice is benzyl penicillin; alternatives are erythromycin or narrow spectrum cephalosporins. Chloramphenicol is active against pneumococci, aminoglycosides *are not*. At least 1 week's treatment is necessary, in severe cases 10–14 days.

Complications
Empyema.   This is often the result of neglect, or suboptimal treatment. It is a difficult problem, as complete drainage of a large purulent effusion is often impossible, and loculation easily leads to persistent low-grade infection, which may only be treatable by surgical drainage.

If empyema develops, it should be drained as thoroughly as possible by needle aspiration, and the patient should be given high doses of antibiotic intravenously. Intrapleural antibiotic is easily inactivated by pus, and is therefore rarely given.

Pericarditis.   This may occur adjacent to infected lung or pleura. Signs are rising jugular venous pressure, falling blood pressure, and central chest pain which often changes with posture. Chest X-ray shows an enlarging heart shadow if an effusion develops. The principles of treatment are as for empyema but the risks of pericardial aspiration are considerable. If aspiration becomes necessary it is best carried out by an experienced operator.

Coincident septicaemia or meningitis.   These demand high-dose intravenous treatment (see Chapters 9 and 10).

Caution.   Signs in the chest X-ray may take some weeks to resolve. Persisting opacity does not usually indicate persisting infection, once the patient appears well.

Prevention
A pneumococcal vaccine has recently become available. It contains polysaccharide antigens of the 14 most common pneumococcal serotypes, and is effective in reducing chest infections in those with predispositions such as sickle cell disease and chronic bronchitis.

It is somewhat less effective in immunosuppressed individuals, and ineffective in infants below age 6–12 months.

Staphylococcal pneumonia

Epidemiology
This is due to *Staphylococcus aureus*, often resident on the skin and in the external nares. Staphylococci may infect the lungs after a previous viral infection, or after treatment of bronchitis with amoxycillin or tetracycline (which are not active against most staphylococci). Pneumonia is common in staphylococcal septicaemia (see Chapter 10)

Clinical features
The features of the underlying condition are accompanied by cough, shortness of breath and yellowish purulent sputum. The chest X-ray shows nodular opacities which vary very much in size and which may cavitate to become abscesses (Fig. 9). Emphyema or a pleural abscess may also develop. The white cell count may remain below 10×10^9/l for a few days, but will then rise. There is always a neutrophilia of 80–95%.

Diagnosis
Sputum and blood culture will provide a definitive diagnosis. The chest

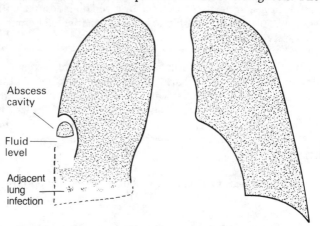

Abscess cavity

Fluid level

Adjacent lung infection

Fig. 9.   Large lung abscess in a case of staphylococcal pneumonia.

X-ray and clinical situation often provide sufficient clues for initial treatment to be started pending cultural information.

Treatment
Penicillinase-resistant antibiotics, such as cloxacillin, flucloxacillin or cephalosporins are the drugs of choice. Fusidic acid is also excellent but should generally be given with another drug as staphylococci can readily become resistant to it. Aminoglycosides are also effective.

Treatment should be given intramuscularly or intravenously for at least 1 week, depending on response.

Caution. *Klebsiella pneumonia* infection, due to *Klebs. pneumoniae*, can complicate chronic chest disease. It produces segmental pneumonia with abscess formation, and the sputum is often brown. Sputum culture will reveal the organism, which is a Gram-negative rod. It is a member of the enterobacteriaceae. Some klebsiellae are sensitive to co-trimoxazole, otherwise aminoglycosides, or very wide-spectrum penicillins or cephalosporins must be used.

Aspiration pneumonia and abscesses

Aspiration of vomitus or secretions into the bronchial tree often results in bronchitis or bronchopneumonia with a tendency to abscess formation. In recumbent patients the infection tends to occur in the apex of a lower lobe. Aspiration of gastric acid produces widespread lung damage and infection (Mendelson's syndrome).

Treatment is with intravenous hydrocortisone to reduce inflammation, and with antibiotics depending on the result of sputum culture as a mixture of organisms is often involved. Ampicillin/cloxacillin combinations, erythromycin or cefuroxime are often useful. Large abscesses sometimes require needle aspiration, but they will often drain spontaneously via the bronchi.

Pertussis (whooping cough)

Epidemiology
This severe respiratory infection spreads by droplet transmission and causes considerable morbidity in children. Adults can be affected, but are less susceptible to severe respiratory complications. In infants, who may acquire it from older sibs, it is a dangerous disease with a significant mortality. The pool of *Bordetella pertussis*, the causative organism, probably exists in schoolchildren. Other organisms, including *B. parapertussis*, adenoviruses, respiratory syncytial virus and influenza viruses are associated with a minority of cases.

Clinical features
After 7–14 days' incubation period the child develops a catarrhal illness with a cough. Over the next week or two the coughs become grouped into paroxysms, first of five or ten, and then 20 or more, often precipitated by feeding or slight external stimulation. The string of sharp coughs changes to grunts, and then gasps as the vital capacity is exhausted, and cyanosis may develop. Some of the paroxysms end in a vomit, and many end with a sustained inspiratory cry (the whoop) as the air is inspired through the narrow glottis.

Mechanical effects of the severe cough can produce subconjunctival or intraocular haemorrhage, or even subdural haemorrhage, as well as irritation of the throat and fraenum of the tongue. Bronchial damage can lead to bronchiectasis. Consolidation due to alveolitis, aspiration or secondary bacterial infection can be fatal in babies and small children. Anoxia and infection can produce encephalopathy and potentially fatal apnoeic attacks.

Illness is prolonged; the cough usually worsens for 2–3 weeks and remains static for another week or two before gradually improving. The whoop may recur with subsequent simple infections for several months after recovery.

Diagnosis
The triad of paroxysmal cough, whoop and vomiting is usually diagnostic. *B. pertussis* is present in bronchial secretions from a few days before the catarrhal illness to 10 days or so after the cough begins. It can be recovered from a pernasal swab taken immediately after a paroxysm, or from an agar plate held 15cm (6 inches) from the coughing child's mouth (cough plate).

By the time the cough is established, the white cell count is usually raised, and comprises 70–80% lymphocytes, a useful sign in late diagnosis.

Treatment
No antibiotic treatment will alter the course of established disease, and it is doubtful whether antibiotic prophylaxis is effective, though some feel that erythromycin may be useful in this respect. Equally, sedatives and antitussives have a limited effect on the cough, and could endanger the airway by causing drowsiness; they should be used only with great care.

The main treatment is non-specific, including clearing mucus from the pharynx, holding the child head-down during attacks to prevent aspiration of vomitus, and feeding carefully and often to avoid provoking paroxysms of coughing.

Aspiration and secondary pneumonia should be treated as already described.

Prevention

Immunization has a significant effect in preventing or ameliorating most attacks. It is valuable in reducing the danger to unimmunized infants, as older sibs who are immunized are less likely to bring the disease into the home. Older children with pertussis should be kept apart from young babies.

Since recent concern about the safety of immunization has markedly reduced acceptance rates, there has been a reappearance of large epidemics of pertussis. In spite of modern medical care, morbidity and mortality have now outstripped that attributed to immunization.

Atypical pneumonias

Epidemiology

These are pneumonias clinically distinct from classical lobar pneumonia, and are caused by organisms which are difficult to isolate in culture. Before serological techniques for diagnosis were widely available their cause was often obscure, and more pathogens associated with atypical pneumonias are likely to be recognized as diagnostic expertise increases (as was the case with legionnaire's disease in the 1970s).

Recognized agents of atypical pneumonia include four main pathogens.

Legionella pneumophila (and other legionellae).   These are fastidious Gram-negative rods which are found in clean stagnant water. Sporadic cases and outbreaks have been related to inhalation (or perhaps consumption) of aerosols from showerheads, cooling towers, air-conditioning plants, moist soil and even cold water taps. This organism is killed by chlorination (hard to achieve in the presence of heat or organic matter) or heating to over 55° C. With an incubation period of 2–10 days, if affects particularly men, smokers and those with pre-existing debilitating diseases.

Mycoplasma pneumoniae.   This, formerly Eaton's agent or pleuro-pneumonia-like organism (PPLO), is a bacterium without a cell wall. It may be a transient resident of the upper respiratory tract, and is acquired by droplet transmission.

Chlamydia psittaci.   Predominantly an intracellular pathogen, this is excreted in the faeces of birds including parrots, budgerigars, ducks, chickens, turkeys and pigeons. It is acquired by inhalation of faeces in aerosols or dust, and affects fanciers, pluckers, packers and breeders of birds, as well as casual contacts.

Coxiella burnetti.   This is the agent of Q fever. Its natural reservoir is in farm animals. Contact, particularly with sheep but also with cows, unpasteurized milk or contaminated straw, is recalled by many patients. It is probably acquired by inhalation or consumption of dust from contaminated areas.

Clinical features

The most common presentation is a feverish illness, myalgia, headache, sweating and constitutional symptoms, with a variable degree of dry cough and abnormality in the chest. The feverish illness may exist alone (if due to *Legionella* it is called Pontiac fever) or be combined with a finding of localized crepitation in the chest or of frank consolidation. There is usually a surprisingly distinct opacity on the chest X-ray, which may be abnormal even when clinical examination seems normal (Fig. 10). Pleurisy and a small pleural effusion sometimes occur. Other variable features include confusion, meningitis, encephalitis, neuropathy, hepatitis and occasional rashes (Fig. 11). *Mycoplasma* infections can also cause pharyngitis, laryngitis and myringitis. Often the illness is self-limiting in 1–3 weeks, but all can be severe, especially when nervous system involvement occurs. Endocarditis is a recognized complication of severe Q fever. Legionnaire's disease is often severe and can be fatal in a week to 10 days if untreated; in particular, cyanosis and a persistently rising blood urea, or bilateral lung involvement, are bad prognostic signs.

The erythrocyte sedimentation rate (ESR) is usually raised above 80mm/hour, particularly in *Mycoplasma* and *Legionella* infections which

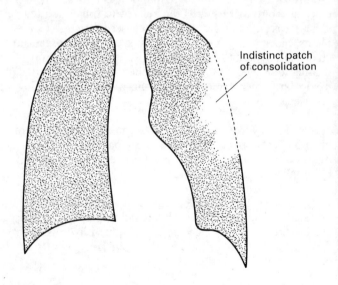

Indistinct patch of consolidation

Fig. 10.   Indistinct lung opacity in a case of atypical pneumonia.

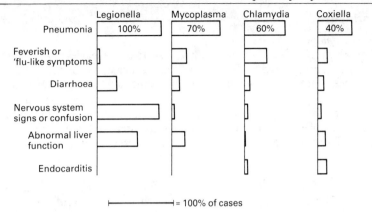

Fig. 11. Approximate incidence of different features in infections due to 'atypical pneumonia' organisms.

are usually associated with a neutrophil leukocytosis. In *Chlamydia* and *Coxiella* infections the white cell count is normal or low.

Diagnosis
As culture requires special facilities, diagnosis is usually based on rising antibody titres in paired sera. Complement fixation tests are reliable except in legionnaire's disease, for which immunofluorescent antibody titres (IFAT) are the best investigations.

Treatment
All of these agents are susceptible to treatment with erythromycin. If legionnaire's disease is suspected (on the basis of pneumonia, diarrhoea, severe confusion, high ESR and history of exposure), treatment should be immediate, and intravenous erythromycin should be given. Alternatives, though less well-tried are rifampicin and chloramphenicol. Treatment should be continued for 10–14 days.

The other atypical pneumonias will often respond to oral erythromycin or tetracycline, though in severe cases, intravenous erythromycin should be given for the first 5–7 days.

Caution. Cytomegalovirus infection can mimic the feverish type of these infections, including the hepatitis, encephalitis and neuropathy, though usually with only a modestly raised ESR (below 60 mm/hour). Inoculation of tissue cultures with early morning urine, throat swabs and genital swabs can reveal the presence of virus. Complement fixation tests show a rising titre of antibodies in the serum. Constant titres of antibody can be seen in the presence of recurrent infection due to activation of latent virus.

Influenza

Epidemiology

The agent of influenza is a myxovirus related to measles virus. Three strains are recognized: A, B and C. Influenza A virus can undergo sudden changes of antigenic structure (antigenic shift) to produce a novel virus type which can spread across the world along routes of communication to produce a pandemic. Influenza B and C change only gradually, so that outbreaks of these occur mainly among children and young people, as adults have often gained immunity through previous exposure.

Clinical features

The incubation period is 2 or 3 days. The illness varies from a mild feverish illness with sore throat or catarrh to a severe infection with alveolitis, lasting for a week or two. Other clinical features, such as meningitis, encephalomyelitis or enteritis are seen in a small number of cases. Adults are more severely affected than children, and tend to develop secondary bacterial infection, particularly with staphylococci.

Diagnosis

The viruses can be isolated in tissue cultures, and rising titres of complement-fixing antibodies appear in paired sera.

Treatment

Bedrest, analgesics and antipyretics are the basis of treatment. Secondary bacterial respiratory infections should be treated with the appropriate antibiotic.

Prevention

There is no reliable means of prevention. Amantadine may ameliorate symptoms if given before or soon after exposure, but is not found useful in normal practice. Influenza vaccines are marketed each year, and afford some protection, which varies with the prevalent strain of virus. Patients with incapacitating respiratory disease, and some health workers are offered immunization, and may benefit from it.

Opportunistic chest infections

These are infections due to organisms which are usually of low pathogenicity, but which invade the lungs of patients with severe immunodeficiency. Leukaemia patients and renal transplant recipients are commonly affected.

Cytomegalovirus

This causes an illness with respiratory distress and a paucity of physical or chest X-ray signs. An indistinct perihilar opacity may be seen on X-ray.

Diagnosis is by tissue culture of sputum or early morning urine, or by complement fixation tests on paired sera. Spontaneous recovery may occur with supportive therapy. Unfortunately the new antiviral agents vidarabine and acyclovir have only slight activity against cytomegalovirus.

Pneumocystis carinii

This is a unicellular organism which causes an illness with severe respiratory distress but few clinical signs. Chest X-ray may show nodular opacities in the hilar and basal areas. Treatment is with co-trimoxazole, which is also often used prophylactically.

Actinomyces spp and Nocardia asteroides

These are filamentous, branching, Gram-positive organisms which produce acute or chronic illness with nodular opacities in the chest X-ray. They are usually sensitive to high-dose penicillins or sulphonamides respectively, but laboratory sensitivity tests should guide therapy. Treatment should ideally be continued for several weeks.

Crytococcus neoformans and Histoplasma capsulatum

These are yeast and fungus organisms. They produce granulomatous infiltration with nodular, or even miliary shadows on the chest X-ray. Cryptococcal meningitis may also occur. Diagnosis is by demonstration of the organism in sputum. There are complement-fixation tests and a histoplasmin skin test for histoplasmosis. Treatment is with intravenous amphotericin, and requires careful supervision because of nausea, hypokalaemia and nephrotoxicity.

Drugs mentioned in this chapter

Drug	Indication	Usage and precautions
Amoxycillin	Acute or chronic bronchitis, secondary chest infections and aspiration infections	Adult dose 250 mg to 1.0 g 8-hourly orally or by intravenous or intramuscular injection; may be combined with cloxacillin or flucloxacillin for secondary infections; child's dose is a quarter to half of adult dose; maculopapular rash is a well-known side-effect
Ampicillin	As above, but less	Adult dose 250 mg to 1.0 g 6-

		well absorbed by mouth	hourly orally or by intravenous or intramuscular injection; child's dose is a quarter to half of adult dose; also causes rash and sometimes diarrhoea
Benzylpenicillin	Drug of choice for pneumococcal pneumonia	Adult dose 600 mg to 2.4 g 6-hourly by intramuscular or intravenous injection or infusion (high doses cannot be given intramuscularly because of severe pain); child's dose is a quarter to half of adult dose
Cephalothin	Alternative to benzylpenicillin; also effective against staphylococci	Adult dose 1.0–2.0 g 4-hourly by intravenous injection; child's dose 12.5 –25 mg/kg 6-hourly
Cefuroxime	Wide spectrum against Gram-positive cocci and *H. influenzae*	Adult dose 750 mg 8-hourly by intramuscular or intravenous injection (this dose can be doubled in severe infections); child's dose 30–100 mg/kg daily in divided doses
Cloxacillin or Flucloxacillin	Active against *Staph. aureus*	Adult dose 250 mg to 1.0 g 6-hourly orally or by intramuscular or intravenous injection; child's dose is a quarter to half of adult dose
Co-trimoxazole	Wide-spectrum; some anti-staphylococcal action	Fixed combination of one part trimethoprim to five parts sulphamethoxazole; adult dose 960 mg 12-hourly orally; child's dose 120–480 mg 12-hourly
	Pneumocystis carinii prophylaxis in chronic bronchitis or mucoviscidosis	The above dose may be doubled; adult dose 960 mg at night; child's dose 120–480 mg at night (prolonged sulphonamide dosage can cause rashes)
Erythromycin	Drug of choice in atypical pneumonias; alternative to benzylpenicillin	Adult dose 300–500 mg 6-hourly intravenously; child's dose 30–60 mg/kg daily in four doses (can be given orally in mild mycoplasmal disease: adult dose 500 mg 6-hourly, child's dose 125–250 mg 6-hourly)
Fusidic acid	Antistaphylococcal	Available as sodium fusidate;

	agent (must *always* be combined with another drug to avoid emergence of resistant staphs	adult dose 500 mg 8-hourly orally; may be given 6-hourly by intravenous injection; absorption is equally good by either route; can cause gastritis (helped by antacids) and severe thrombophlebitis (when intravenous dosage must be used); child's dose 175–350 mg 8-hourly; overdosage causes reversible cholestatic jaundice
Hydrocortisone	For relief of severe mucosal oedema	Adult dose 200–500 mg by intravenous bolus injection; child's dose 50–100 mg intravenously
Tetracyclines	Acute or chronic bronchitis in domiciliary practice, atypical pneumonias (*except* legionnaire's disease); prophylaxis in chronic bronchitis	Adult dose of oxytetracycline is 250–500 mg 6-hourly orally; tetracyclines are not given to children as they stain and damage growing teeth and bones; many tetracyclines exacerbate renal impairment; usually doxycycline 100 mg at night orally; this agent does not affect renal function

5

Intestinal Infections and Food Poisoning

Intestinal infection results from the consumption of organisms which become established in the bowel and attack the mucosa (Fig. 12). Many agents are transmitted by faecal–oral spread either directly by the hands, by flies and cockroaches, on food prepared by hand, or in water contaminated by sewage.

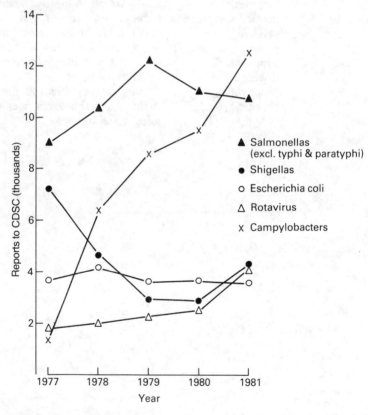

Fig. 12. Common gastrointestinal pathogens: changing trends, England, Wales and Northern Ireland.

Food poisoning is the illness which follows consumption of food contaminated by bacteria, bacterial toxins or toxic chemicals. Some enteric infections are transmitted by food, and some food poisoning may result from faecal–oral contamination; for instance salmonellae are usually regarded as food poisoning agents, though they can be acquired by faecal-oral transmission as well. Conversely, food is often the source of *Campylobacter* enteritis. Because of this overlap of nomenclature, some definitions may appear slightly arbitrary. Other common terms are *gastroenteritis*, a syndrome of liquid diarrhoea and vomiting usually associated with small bowel infections, and *dysentery*, a syndrome of diarrhoea with mucus and sometimes blood, usually the result of large bowel infection and mucosal excoriation.

Symptoms and signs of enteric infections
Fever.   This is very variable. In some conditions, such as severe dysentery it is always present, while in others, such as *Escherichia coli* or *Salmonella* enteritis it may only be present at the onset of disease. Some patients have no fever by the time of presentation, but this does not exclude a diagnosis of infection. A continuing fever is often a sign that early improvement is not to be expected.

Abdominal pain.   This is also a variable feature. In salmonellosis it is often trivial or absent. In dysentery and clostridial food poisoning it can be severe, central and colicky, and is usually associated with episodes of diarrhoea. In amoebic or *Campylobacter* infections there may be constant generalized abdominal pain, and even rebound tenderness. In these circumstances the presence of bowel sounds, which are usually hyperactive, and of diarrhoea will reassure the physician that peritonitis and ileus are unlikely diagnoses.

Caution.   Surgical conditions sometimes produce diarrhoea and abdominal pain. Common problems include early appendicitis, especially in children, gynaecological infections, and partial bowel obstruction due to faecal impaction or neoplasm, with spurious diarrhoea. It is very important to re-examine the patient at intervals for the appearance of localizing signs.

Vomiting.   Except in viral gastroenteritis, when it seldom lasts for more than a day or two, vomiting alone is unusual in enteric infections. More often than not it accompanies the first hours or days of diarrhoea, or precedes the diarrhoea by a few hours.

If vomiting occurs alone, alternative diagnoses should be considered, including ear and vestibular disease, brainstem disorders, uraemia and other metabolic disorders, drugs, bowel obstruction, and pregnancy. Vomiting with severe abdominal pain may be due to pancreatitis, biliary or ureteric colic, peptic ulcer, aortic aneurism or myocardial infarction.

Diarrhoea.   This is a loosely applied term which means the passage of too frequent or unusually loose stools. The nature of the diarrhoea may be characteristic of a particular type of illness, so it is important to examine the patient's stools. Features to look for are colour, presence of mucus or blood, presence of worms or segments of tapeworms, and the bulk of the stool (very bulky stools are seen in malabsorption and in some parasitic diseases). The fluid part of the stool is most likely to contain the pathogens, and this should be sent to the laboratory for examination.

Caution.   Watery diarrhoea may be seen in irritable bowel disease, inflammatory bowel disease, drug reactions, laxative abuse and thyrotoxicosis. Blood may be present in cases with inflammatory bowel disease, diverticular disease and ischaemic colitis. Blood and mucus may be seen in inflammatory disease of the colon, and neoplastic diseases. Finally, it is always wise to be sure that a patient's diarrhoea is not melaena!

The abdominal X-ray.   During enteric infection, the patient's bowel is usually full of gas and fluid faeces. An erect abdominal X-ray will therefore show many fluid levels, and this must not be taken as evidence of obstruction unless there is supporting clinical evidence such as absent bowel sounds or constipation. A plain abdominal X-ray will be useful if the differential diagnosis is inflammatory bowel disease, as it can reveal toxic dilatation of the colon.

Barium enema examination is indicated when patients have persisting diarrhoea with no detectable pathogens in the stool.

Dehydration.   This is often the most serious management problem in cases of enteric infection. Those at particular risk are babies, whose blood volume is small compared with the volume of diarrhoea stools, and the elderly, who may have very poor cardiovascular reserve and be unable to compensate for even a small reduction in blood volume. In cholera and other severe diarrhoeal illnesses, even previously fit patients may be unable to tolerate fluid losses of up to 20 litres per day.

Danger signs are sunken eyes, stiff and dry skin, listlessness, tachycardia, lack of urine output and falling blood pressure. Babies may be weighed, several times daily if necessary, to detect fluid loss. A steady weight indicates adequate fluid balance.

The commonest electrolyte abnormality is a lowered plasma sodium level, which in severe cases can be well below 120mmol/l. The plasma potassium level may also be low. A combination of infection, starvation and electrolyte imbalance sometimes results in severe acidosis. The haemoglobin and blood urea levels rise in severe dehydration.

Treatment of dehydration in enteric infections.   The diarrhoea in enteric infections is often due, in part at least, to the osmotic effect of small peptides and sugars which remain unabsorbed in the bowel lumen. Lactose is a major contributor to this, as the lactase mucosal enzyme system is usually the first to suffer in enteric infections. The first step in treatment, therefore, is to stop milk feeds and solid foods, and to give clear fluids instead.

Another mechanism of diarrhoea is that of hypersecretion by the mucosal cells when they are affected by the toxins of organisms such as cholera vibrios or toxigenic *E. coli*. Fortunately the sodium and glucose absorption mechanisms are unaffected, so that oral fluids containing these substances will be absorbed. Sodium and glucose absorption are interdependent, so a certain glucose concentration aids maximum absorption of sodium and water (Table 4). The high concentration of

Table 4. Some useful rehydration solutions

Solution	Electrolytes (mmol/litre)					
	Sodium	Chloride	Potassium	Bicarbonate	Calcium	Glucose
Oral solution						
Solution recommended by the World Health Organization	90	80	20	30	—	110
Sodium chloride and dextrose oral powder compound (BNF)	35	37	20	18	—	200
Half-strength Hartmann's solution	65.5	55.5	2.5	14.5	1.0	—
Intravenous solution						
Dextrose 4%, saline 0.18% with potassium 5 mmol/l	30	35	5	—	—	—
Hartmann's (compound sodium lactate) solution	131	111	5	29	2	—
Ringer's solution	147	155	4	—	2	—

NOTE: The intravenous preparations 'Paediatric Electrolyte Solution®' and Darrow's solution both contain 35 mmol/l potassium, and cannot therefore be infused rapidly.

The solutions with the higher sodium concentrations are ideal for rehydration, but the lower sodium solutions are best for maintenance hydration as they are less likely to cause sodium overload.

Breast milk, or diluted breast milk can be used for maintenance of hydration.

potassium ensures passive absorption of this ion down a concentration gradient. Fluids such as this may be given freely by bottle, cup or spoon feeding. These suggested values are not critical; sucrose can be used instead of glucose with a little loss of efficacy, but too much of any sugar will result in osmotic diarrhoea. Commercial powders are available in sachets for making up in boiled or sterile water.

If oral rehydration is unsuccessful and the patient fails to regain his normal weight and the urine output or the blood pressure falls, then intravenous rehydration is indicated. Suitable fluids are shown in Table 4. Normal saline (0.9% or 150 mmol/l) may provide a rather excessive concentration of sodium for normal purposes.

Minimum fluid requirements in healthy individuals vary from 100 ml/kg daily in infants to 40 or 50 ml/kg daily in adults. Initial rapid infusion of 200–250 ml for babies, or a litre or more in 15 minutes for adults, can be used to replace severe fluid loss. Thereafter allowance for the loss in diarrhoea stools must be added to the basic requirement.

Caution.   Rapid infusion of fluids in the aged can easily result in severe pulmonary oedema. Even with most cautious rehydration this cannot be avoided in some patients, in whom diarrhoea is then a life-threatening disorder.

Hypernatraemic dehydration.   This unusual condition tends to occur in babies aged about a year, and is often associated with the use of high-sodium or insufficiently diluted milk feeds. The child does not appear dehydrated, but is irritable. He has reddened conjunctivae, and may have fits. The plasma sodium is often in the range of 150–160 mmol/l, and uraemia or acidosis may also exist.

Too-rapid dilution of the plasma will result in cerebral oedema and fits. Cautious replacement of fluid loss with normal saline, or one of the compound sodium lactate solutions, is given until the urine output is adequate. This is followed by the gradual introduction of more dilute fluids, such as half-normal saline in small aliquots. If convulsions occur they may be controlled with small intramuscular doses of diazepam, or with oral phenobarbitone or phenytoin. The prognosis of hypernatraemic dehydration is less good than that of other types.

Postinfectious diarrhoea.   When milk feeds are reintroduced after an episode of diarrhoea in babies, loose stools may recur because of persisting lactase deficiency. If severe this problem can be overcome by feeding a low-lactose milk mixture such as Galactomin 19 or Pregestimil until ordinary feeds can be tolerated. Occasionally more extreme malabsorption of proteins and fats requires special dietary measures, devised with the help of an experienced dietician. After severe dysentery some adults can benefit from a milk-free diet for a short time.

Use of drugs to alleviate symptoms. Severe diarrhoea rarely responds to antidiarrhoeal agents. Kaolin mixture, codeine phosphate, loperamide or diphenoxylate–atropine tablets (Lomotil) are sometimes helpful in moderate cases, and the atropinic action of the last two may alleviate distressing colic.

Caution. Atropinic drugs easily cause toxicity in small children and are therefore contraindicated.

Phenothiazines such as promethazine or prochlorperazine (Stemetil), and metoclopramide (Maxolon, Primperan) are effective in the treatment of vomiting. It should be borne in mind that they are mildly sedative.

Viral gastroenteritis

Epidemiology
Rotaviruses are the commonest cause of viral gastroenteritis in children below age 2, but can also cause disease in older children and adults. They probably spread mainly by the faecal–oral route, as large numbers are excreted in the faeces of affected patients. Extensive outbreaks have been reported in paediatric and neonatal wards. Caliciviruses and astroviruses are similar in appearance, and are probably transmitted in the same way. Adenoviruses have also been associated with some outbreaks of diarrhoea in children. In these outbreaks there is evidence for both faecal–oral and airborne transmission. There is now evidence that some small, unnamed viruses can be transmitted by food, particularly soft fruit and shellfish.

Clinical features
After an incubation period of about a day, a mildly feverish illness occurs, with watery diarrhoea and a variable amount of vomiting. Children often also have a slight nasal discharge. The illness seldom lasts more than 5 days.

Winter vomiting disease, which has been associated with calcivirus infection, usually lasts for about 2 days, with profuse vomiting on the first day and fatigue on the second. Several members of a family may rapidly be affected. Diarrhoea is trivial or absent. Moderate degrees of dehydration can occur in these viral infections.

Diagnosis
Rotavirus and calicivirus particles can be demonstrated in the stool by electron microscopy. Adenovirus can be isolated from stool specimens by tissue culture. Rotavirus antigen in stools is detectable by Enzyme-Linked ImmunoSorbent Assay (ELISA)

Treatment
This is symptomatic and is mainly directed at maintenance of correct fluid balance.

Escherichia coli gastroenteritis

Epidemiology
Escherichia coli is a resident of the bowel, of which many O (somatic) and
H (flagellar) serotypes are recognized. Altogether 17 of the O serotypes
have been shown to be associated with gastroenteritis in infants. They are
known as enteropathogenic or enteropathic *E. coli* (EPEC) and are responsible for sporadic disease and for epidemics in nurseries and hospital
wards. Some serotypes of *E. coli* produce a toxin, similar in action to
cholera toxin. These are known as enterotoxigenic *E. coli* (ETEC), and
are thought to be responsible for many cases of 'traveller's diarrhoea'.
Other strains which adhere to mucosal cells or invade them are known as
invasive (EIEC) or adhesive (EAEC) types and their clinical significance
is a subject for study.
   Transmission of *E. coli* gastroenteritis is by the faecal–oral route, and
is particularly likely when more than one infant is attended by the
same nurse.

Clinical features
The incubation period is about 2 days. Fever, vomiting and diarrhoea can
all be prominent features of the disease, which may be mild and self-
limiting or severe and prolonged. Clinical distinction from other types of
gastroenteritis is not possible. In severe cases dehydration is a major
problem and can lead to fatalities. Lactose malabsorption is common
after such illness.

Diagnosis
This is based on isolation of *E. coli* from stool cultures and serological distinction from non-pathogenic strains.

Treatment
This is concerned mainly with the maintenance of fluid and electrolyte
balance. When the diarrhoea has subsided, feeding is begun with a
quarter-strength milk mixture, and the strength of feed is increased daily
as long as diarrhoea does not recur. If dilute milk feeds cause recurrence
of diarrhoea, a low lactose feed should be substituted until milk is
again tolerated.

Salmonella enteritis

Epidemiology
Often referred to as 'food poisoning', salmonella enteritis is the commonest food-borne infection. It can be acquired from all kinds of meat
and fowl and their offal, sometimes from fish, and from food contaminated by handlers. The cavity of the meat is contaminated by bowel-
originating salmonellae. The centre of a large joint or fowl may remain

frozen after hurried thawing. The resulting inadequate cooking is a common cause of salmonellosis outbreaks. Faecal–oral spread is also common between farm herds, between humans, and from one to the other. Pet animals including reptiles such as snakes and terrapins can be symptomless excretors of salmonellae and provide a source of infection for their keepers.

Clinical features
The incubation period is from 12 to 24 hours, but can occasionally be longer. Some people acquire the organism and excrete it in the stools without developing symptoms.

Most patients have abrupt onset of diarrhoea, initially accompanied by mild fever and a variable amount of vomiting. The duration of diarrhoea is usually a day or two longer than that of the fever. The illness often resolves in 2–5 days, but is sometimes prolonged to 2 weeks or more.

The excretor state. Many patients continue to excrete the organism for a few days, or sometimes weeks, after clinical cure. Follow-up is usually required in excretors who work in schools, nurseries or the food and dairy trade, as they should be 'cleared' before returning to work. Three consecutive negative stool cultures are usually required for this purpose by the MOEH concerned, though it is rarely necessary for the patient to remain in hospital for clearance unless social circumstances compel him to do so (for instance in the case of a child from an orphanage, or an adult from a residential institution). The likelihood of cross-infection from an excretor is much reduced when diarrhoea has ceased. Prolonged excretion of salmonellae is rare in otherwise healthy individuals.

Caution: achlorhydric patients. Patients who lack gastric acid because of pernicious anaemia or previous gastric surgery have greatly reduced natural defence against salmonellae, and easily contract severe illness from apparently insignificant challenge. They often have profuse watery diarrhoea and a grossly raised blood urea level. Positive blood cultures indicating transient bacteraemia rather than septicaemia are the rule, but if they are persistently positive parenteral antibiotic treatment may have to be considered.

Caution: sickle cell disease. Patients with sickle cell disease can develop salmonella osteomyelitis even without clinical evidence of bacteraemia.

Diagnosis
The organism can be cultured from the diarrhoea stool. Food remaining from a suspect meal, a food handler or an animal contact may also produce positive cultures.

A neutrophil leukocytosis is usual in the acute stage.

Treatment
Antibiotics are contraindicated in simple enteritis, because they do not affect the clinical features and they often prolong the excretor state. Attention to fluid and electrolyte balance is usually all that is needed. In the rare cases with severe disease and persistently positive blood cultures treatment with chloramphenicol is indicated, as for enteric fevers.

Campylobacter enteritis

Epidemiology
Campylobacters are Gram-negative, microaerophilic bacteria which are found in the bowel of animals and birds. Common sources of infection in man include chicken, undercooked beef, unpasteurized milk, domestic pets and water contaminated by animal or bird faeces. Person-to-person transmission is rare.

Clinical features
The incubation period is 2–8 days, often about 3 days, and it ends with rapid onset of fever, malaise, headache and abdominal pain. After a few hours diarrhoea begins. This is usually watery and in a minority of cases it is bloody. Abdominal pain is a major feature of the illness, and because it tends to be constant and generalized, often with associated slight rebound tenderness, it may suggest a surgical diagnosis. Hyperactive bowel sounds and the early onset of diarrhoea will help to resolve this problem.

Occasionally, illness is prolonged with bloody diarrhoea and abdominal colic persisting for weeks. A diagnosis of ulcerative colitis may then be considered, and mucosal biopsy or even sigmoidoscopy may appear to support this. However if the stool cultures produce a growth of *Campylobacter spp.*, appropriate treatment will often terminate the illness.

The asymptomatic carrier state is rare.

Diagnosis
The organisms can be cultured from the diarrhoea stools. There is usually a neutrophil leukocytosis.

Treatment
Most cases will recover in 3–5 days with only supportive treatment. Severe or prolonged illness will respond to a 3 or 4 days' course of oral erythromycin.

Cases of campylobacter enteritis with septicaemia have been described in debilitated children. Parenteral erythromycin is the treatment of choice in these cases.

Bacillary dysenteries

Epidemiology
The bacillary dysenteries fall into two loosely separated epidemiological groups each consisting of two *Shigella* species:

(1) *Sh. sonnei* and *Sh. boydii*, which are relatively common in developed countries as well as the less-developed, and which often cause outbreaks in schools and children's institutions where spread is by faecal–oral transmission;

(2) *Sh. flexneri* and *Sh. dysenteriae*, which are rarely contracted in developed countries, but which tend to spread by faecal contamination of water and food in Asian, African and some South American countries.

Clinical features
Shigella sonnei and *Sh. boydii* both tend to produce self-limiting disease which begins, after an incubation period of 2 or 3 days, with sudden onset of high fever. During the duration of the fever, children in particular may suffer from delirium, meningism or febrile convulsions. All investigations are normal except for the presence of a neutrophil leukocytosis. After 6–12 hours diarrhoea commences and the temperature soon falls. The diarrhoea is watery, sometimes with small amounts of blood and mucus, and is associated with colicky abdominal pain. Illness usually lasts no more than 5 or 6 days.

Sh. flexneri and *Sh. dysenteriae* have a similar onset but, instead of falling when the diarrhoea begins, the temperature continues to fluctuate widely. Abdominal pain may be severe at times and, as colonic ulceration progresses, increasing amounts of blood mingle with the mucus in the stools. Illness can continue for weeks with rapidly increasing exhaustion, anaemia and wasting.

Diagnosis
The clinical features may suggest the diagnosis. Confirmation depends on the isolation of the organism from diarrhoea stools. Rarely a positive blood culture is obtained; this usually represents a chance finding of bacteraemia and requires no specific treatment. Asymptomatic carriage may persist for a few weeks after recovery.

Treatment
The milder types rarely require other than symptomatic treatment. *Sh. flexneri* dysentery will usually respond to a 1-week course of oral trimethoprim, but is often resistant to ampicillin or amoxycillin. *Sh. dysenteriae* is likely to respond to ampicillin given orally. If *Sh. sonnei* infection requires specific treatment, oral streptomycin is an additional alternative to ampicillin or trimethoprim.

Yersinia infection

Epidemiology
Yersinia enterocolitica and *Y. pseudotuberculosis* are Gram-negative rods widespread in soil and water. They can also be recovered from the faeces of some farm animals. The route of transmission to man is either by faecal–oral spread from man or animal, or by contaminated water. They are not often included in the list of enteric pathogens sought by routine laboratories, and case numbers are therefore small.

Clinical features
Three main clinical presentations are recognized.

Enteritis.   Yersinia infections are estimated to be associated with up to 5% of childhood gastroenteritis cases in Europe.

'Appendicular' syndromes.   These usually occur in older children or adolescents, and include terminal ileitis, sometimes with mesenteric adenitis.

'Reactive' states.   These are thought to be related to the immune response to yersinia infections, and include erythema nodosum, large joint arthritis, and, rarely, glomerulonephritis and thyroiditis.
   Septicaemia sometimes occurs in children, particularly those with haemochromatosis or thalassaemia.

Diagnosis
In acute illness the organism can be recovered from stool cultures. Rising titres of antibodies may also be found in paired sera.

Treatment
Specific treatment may not be required, especially in simple enteritis. Otherwise laboratory sensitivity tests should guide the choice of antibiotic. Oral tetracycline is often useful.

Cholera

Epidemiology
Toxigenic strains of *Vibrio cholerae* can exist in water, particularly the stagnant water of ponds and canals, and will cause disease if ingested by man. The reservoir of infection probably exists among sick people, and a lesser number of asymptomatic carriers. The classical biotype of *V. cholerae* is slowly being superseded by the El Tor biotype which survives longer in adverse conditions, and is more likely to exist in asymptomatic carriers.
   Non-cholera vibrios are natural inhabitants of stagnant and brackish

water, and some cause disease in man. *V. parahaemolyticus* is found in estuaries and may be eaten with shellfish, resulting in a sharp attack of diarrhoea and abdominal colic.

Clinical features
After an incubation period of a few hours to a few days, illness begins with diarrhoea. Cholera toxin causes the bowel mucosa to secrete large amounts of fluid which appear as the typical 'rice water' stool. Illness varies from mild to fulminant, in which 20 or more litres of stool are produced daily with little or no interval between evacuations. Achlorhydria predisposes to severe symptoms after even minimal exposure. Fever and abdominal pain are not normally a major part of the illness. Dehydration and electrolyte depletion are an immediate and continuing problem in severe cases.

Diagnosis
Vibrio cholerae can be isolated from the diarrhoea stool. Culture for vibrios is not carried out routinely in laboratories in Western countries, and it should therefore be specifically requested if cholera is suspected.

Treatment
The immediate requirement is skilful management of fluid and electrolyte replacement. Oral oxytetracycline will usually reduce the severity and duration of the illness, and is also of use in the treatment of asymptomatic carriers. It is also effective in prophylaxis and offers a useful adjunct to the currently available vaccines when heavy exposure is anticipated.

Follow-up
The families and other close contacts of patients should be investigated for the presence of a carrier state. In Britain it is customary to obtain six consecutive negative stool samples before releasing the patient from surveillance.

Amoebiasis

Epidemiology
Entamoeba histolytica is a parasitic protozoan. It survives well in the colon of man where it may cause disease. Trophozoites and cysts may be passed in the stool, and the cysts are infectious if they are ingested. Transmission is usually via drinking water, contaminated with faeces from asymptomatic carriers or individuals with amoebiasis. Infection is most common in tropical regions.

Clinical features
Intestinal amoebiasis. This is the commonest form of amoebiasis. Inges-

tion of *E. histolytica* cysts is followed by a variable incubation period, depending partly on the size of the challenge. Some individuals then become asymptomatic carriers, and pass cysts in the stool. Others develop chronic relapsing diarrhoea, which may be associated with the slow development of mucosal masses of granulation tissue, called amoebomas. These masses occur most commonly in the caecum and ascending colon, and may be taken for carcinomas on barium enema examination. This chronic state is a frequent finding in endemic areas. Finally, some patients develop severe or fulminating dysentery with fever, abdominal pain, and diarrhoea with blood and mucus. Again the caecum is the site of most inflammation and ulceration, so that right iliac fossa pain is prominent. Perforation of the bowel can lead to faecal and amoebic peritonitis in the most severe cases.

There is usually a neutrophil leukocytosis in those patients who have symptoms.

Hepatic amoebiasis.   Severe amoebic dysentery may be associated with jaundice and hepatocellular disturbance of liver function tests. This is called amoebic hepatitis and appears to be reactive rather than due to invasion of the liver by amoebae. It responds to treatment of the dysentery.

Amoebic abscess of the liver is a more serious problem which rarely occurs without previous amoebic dysentery. High swinging fever, painful enlargement of the liver and marked neutrophil leukocytosis are the signs. Ultrasound or isotope scan of the liver usually shows a single abscess which is most often in the right lobe. A large abscess may 'point' at the chest or abdominal wall. Needle aspiration produces pinkish-brown 'anchovy sauce' pus.

Other types of amoebiasis.   Abscesses may appear in the pleura, lung or pericardium, often by extension from the liver. Necrotic, ulcerated skin lesions with undermined edges sometimes occur due to faecal inoculation in excoriated skin.

Diagnosis

Cysts or trophozoites may be seen in stool smears from patients with intestinal amoebiasis. If they are adherent to the rectal mucosa they can sometimes be seen in smears made from material rubbed off the mucosa by an examining glove. Only fresh specimens are suitable for this type of examination; they should be sent to the laboratory in a thermos flask, to avoid rapid cooling.

If amoebae cannot be found in the stool, they may be found on histological examination of biopsies from the ulcerated mucosa. Fluid from abscesses rarely contains amoebae, which adhere to the abscess wall.

Serological diagnosis.   Patients with dysentery or extraintestinal amoebiasis quickly acquire a positive fluorescent antibody test (FAT). As the FAT titre falls when infection is terminated, a high or rising titre may be interpreted as indicating active infection. Other types of antibodies can be detected over a different time-course.

Treatment
The treatment of choice for both dysentery and extraintestinal amoebiasis is metronidazole, given orally or intravenously as is expedient. Moderately large liver abscesses will resolve without drainage, others may require repeated needle aspiration. Left-lobe liver abscesses may require surgical drainage. Treatment should be continued for 7–14 days, or until any abscess has resolved. Chloroquine enters the wall of liver abscesses, and is a useful additional drug if metronidazole alone is ineffective.

   Asymptomatic cyst-passers or mild intestinal cases respond less well to metronidazole, and may require treatment with a 10-day course of a luminal amoebicide such as diloxanide, either alone or following a course of metronidazole.

Follow-up.
Stool examination should be repeated 1 month after treatment to detect persistent infection. Further treatment with a luminal amoebicide is indicated in carriers.

Giardiasis

Epidemiology
Giardia lamblia is a flagellate protozoan which adheres to the duodenal mucosa by means of a ventral sucker. It forms cysts which are passed in the stool and which will infect others if ingested. The usual source of infection is water contaminated by the faeces of asymptomatic or symptomatic cyst passers. It is possible that dogs may harbour the organism. Giardiasis is a worldwide infection, but is most common in hot countries.

Clinical features
These probably depend on the number of pathogens in the bowel. Asymptomatic carriage with intermittent passage of cysts is common. Symptomatic infection often causes diarrhoea and flatulence which is particularly troublesome in the morning and improves by evening. Severe infection causes a malabsorption (sprue) syndrome with bulky, greasy stools and significant weight loss.

Diagnosis
Typical cysts may be seen in stool preparations, but this is not always the case. If the diagnosis is strongly suspected, it may be proved by aspiration of duodenal contents, or microscopic examination of a soft string which can be swallowed in a capsule and later retrieved. Duodenal biopsy may also reveal the organism, attached to the sides of the villi.

Treatment
The treatment of choice is oral metronidazole, given for 1 week or, in larger dosage, for 3 days. Relapse is not uncommon, and should be treated with a further course of metronidazole.

Trichinosis

This is a rare but potentially serious disease caused by an invasive nematode, *Trichinella spiralis*. Infection is caused by ingestion of viable cysts in undercooked pork (or bear meat). After 2 days incubation abdominal pain, nausea and diarrhoea occur. Eosinophilia is common.

After a further day or two, developing worms leave the bowel and travel via the circulation to the muscles, where they encyst. This process may continue for a month or more producing myalgia, fever, increasing eosinophilia, and allergic manifestations including urticaria and facial oedema. Occasionally the worms enter the nervous system, causing meningism, cerebral irritation or polyneuritis. This is a life-threatening situation.

Diagnosis is made by finding a positive fluorescent antibody test or complement fixation test on serological examination. Muscle biopsy may reveal the presence of cysts.

Treatment is with oral thiabendazole. Prednisolone may be given to alleviate allergic manifestations or cerebral irritation.

Toxic food poisoning

Any time which elapses between the preparation and consumption of food will allow the multiplication of micro-organisms in the food, and elaboration of their toxins. This process occurs more quickly if the food is kept warm.

There are also toxins present in some foods which are not produced by microbial organisms but are ingested and retained by food animals, elaborated by plants or produced by spoilage of food.

Staphylococcal food poisoning
Staphylococcus aureus is introduced into food from the skin or nasopharynx of food handlers. It commonly contaminates sandwiches, cakes, cheese dishes and sweetmeats prepared by hand. It can produce several different enterotoxins, which resist brief cooking.

After 2–6 hours incubation period, severe vomiting and sometimes diarrhoea occur. Dehydration can be profound, but the illness seldom lasts more than 2 days.

Staph. aureus can be cultured from specimens of vomitus, and the organism and toxins may be found in leftover food.

Bacillus cereus

Spores of this aerobic organism exist in soil, vegetables and cereals. They survive boiling and later germinate in kept food (often in boiled rice kept for frying) and produce enterotoxin. Two different *B. cereus* toxins are known to produce two types of illness.

The incubation period is usually from 1 to 6 hours. The illness produced is similar to staphylococcal food poisoning, but the organism is found in the patient's faeces as well as in the contaminated food. *B. subtilis* is capable of producing similar food poisoning.

A less common diarrhoeal form of illness has an incubation period of 6–16 hours.

Clostridium perfringens (formerly C. welchii)

This organism is widespread in human and animal faeces, raw meats and soil. Spores survive cooking and germinate in the warm, anaerobic interior of meats, stews and gravies.

Organisms are later consumed with the food, and multiply in the bowel, producing an enterotoxin.

The incubation period of 8–22 hours is followed by watery diarrhoea with cramping abdominal pain. The illness may last for 2 or 3 days.

Organisms can be recovered from food or from the patient's faeces.

Clostridium botulinum (botulism)

Spores of *Cl. botulinum* exist in earth and mud. Three main types—A, B and E—affect human beings by contaminating vegetables and fruit, or fish and game. The spores survive all cooking methods except prolonged pressure cooking. The spores will only germinate in strictly anaerobic conditions as in canned, bottled or oil-preserved foods, and are inhibited from germinating by the acidity of sweet fruits and most tomatoes. Home-canned or home-bottled vegetables are a common source of outbreaks.

Toxin ingestion may be followed by a brief attack of diarrhoea. The toxin is then absorbed and becomes fixed in the nervous system where, after 18–36 hours it blocks neuromuscular transmission. The patient complains of fatigue, dry mouth, blurred and double vision and increasing difficulty in speaking. Paralysis can progress quite suddenly to the respiratory muscles, though tendon reflexes are retained until a late stage. Constipation is usual.

Diagnosis is based on finding the organism and toxin in food, or toxin in the patient's faeces. Polyvalent antitoxin (effective against types A, B and E) may prevent further toxin activity if given promptly. Antitoxin may also be given prophylactically to others who shared the affected food. If intensive care is available to maintain life, the paralysis will begin a slow recovery after 7–10 days.

Infant botulism.   Infants between the ages of 2 and 6 months (an incidence corresponding exactly to that of 'cot death'), can develop a type of botulism in which large amounts of toxin and organisms are excreted in the stool. The clinical features are the same as in adults, and mild or subclinical cases with only brief feeding difficulty are probably common. Most babies recover without receiving antitoxin. The source of their infection is unknown and, fortunately, their toxic faeces have not presented a public health hazard.

Clostridium difficile
This is the organism whose toxin is associated with pseudomembranous colitis. It is not known how the organism is acquired, but it is usually an opportunistic pathogen in patients whose bowel flora has been altered by antibiotic therapy or by preparation for surgery. The organism and toxin are present in the faeces. Sigmoidoscopic and biopsy features are diagnostic. Treatment is with a 7-day course of oral vancomycin, which may need to be repeated after a 1-week interval.

Non-microbial toxins
Dinoflagellate toxins
In certain parts of the world dinoflagellate plankton multiply greatly in warm weather and colour the sea pink. These organisms contain a toxin which is concentrated in the bodies of shellfish feeding on them. Human beings who eat the contaminated shellfish develop diarrhoea, fatigue and tingling in the fingers. Wise gourmets avoid shellfish during the 'red tide' season.

Scombrotoxin
This is a toxin produced by slight spoilage of scombroid fish (mackerel, tuna and bonito), and occasionally of other fish (sardines, herrings and pilchards). High concentrations of histamine are found in affected fish, and it is likely that scombrotoxin is also an amine. The toxin is not destroyed by boiling, smoking or canning. Poisoning results in diarrhoea, headache, urticaria and flushing, all of which can be ameloriated by treatment with antihistamines.

Bean poisoning
Red kidney beans and, to a lesser extent, haricot and butter beans contain a toxin which is a haemagglutinin. Although soaking the beans removes some toxin, only boiling until the beans are soft will remove it all. Only

four or five undercooked beans are needed to produce a sharp attack of diarrhoea with nausea or vomiting.

Worms and flukes (see Table 5)

Table 5. Some common intestinal worms and flukes

Threadworm (*Enterobius vermicularis*)	Distribution: world-wide Lifecycle: adult worm emerges onto perianal skin at night to deposit eggs; scratching transfers eggs to fingers and they are then ingested to develop in the bowel Diagnosis: eggs can be picked up from anal skin on transparent sticky-tape and viewed under microscope Treatment: piperazine or mebendazole
Whipworm (*Trichuris trichiura*)	Distribution: world-wide Lifecycle: adult worm attaches to colonic mucosa; eggs are passed in faeces and may be ingested or used to fertilize food plants; new adults emerge in colon Diagnosis: eggs visible in faeces smears Treatment: mebendazole or thia-bendazole
Roundworm (*Ascaris lumbricoides*)	Distribution: world-wide Lifecycle: adults inhabit small bowel and eggs are passed in faeces; on ingestion they produce larvae which bore through mucosa and travel in the blood stream to the lungs (causing eosinophilia, cough and CXR opacities —pulmonary eosinophilia); they pass up the trachea, and are swallowed to develop to adulthood in the bowel Large worm loads can cause bowel obstruction Diagnosis: eggs visible in faeces smear Treatment: piperazine, mebendazole
Hookworm (*Ancylostoma duodenale, Necator americanus*)	Distribution: widespread in tropical regions Lifecycle: adults inhabit duodenum and damage mucosa with cutting mouths, causing anaemia; eggs passed in faeces and develop to free-living larvae in damp soil; larvae bore through human skin, causing mild irritation (ground itch) and pass to lungs. They

Strongyloides stercoralis

Cutaneous larva migrans

Tapeworms (commonly *Taenia saginata, T. solium*)

ascend the trachea and are swallowed to infect the gut

Diagnosis: eggs visible in faecal smears

Treatment: mebendazole or thiabendazole

Distribution: particularly tropical Indo-China and South America

Lifecycle: adults inhabit upper small bowel and eggs develop to larvae in faeces; larvae are excreted and can become infectious in damp soil (they can also pursue free-living lifecycles in soil); larvae bore through human skin and travel via alveoli and trachea to bowel; larvae from faeces can bore through bowel wall and reinfect the same host

Diagnosis: larvae visible in faecal smears

Treatment: thiabendazole

This occurs when larvae of animal hookworms enter human skin and migrate aimlessly; penetration of *Strongyloides* larvae from the bowel of an 'immune' host produces the same condition; red tracks are seen in the skin, and there may be urticaria and marked eosinophilia; immunosuppression can result in life-threatening invasive strongyloidiasis

Treated with thiabendazole

Distribution: world-wide

Lifecycle: worm attaches to bowel wall by hooks or suckers on head (scolex); produces segments (proglottides) and eggs; eggs eaten from pasture by cows (*T. saginata*) or pigs (*T. solium*) and hatch in stomach or duodenum; larvae bore through bowel wall and migrate to muscles where they encyst (*T. solium* larvae may leave the bowel of man, if eggs present in duodenum, and cause damaging cysts in brain and muscles—cysticercosis); man eats meat containing cysts (measly meat) and larvae develop into adult worms

Diagnosis: eggs and proglottides seen in faeces

Treatment: niclosamide (if scolex not passed in faeces, later retreatment is needed)

The cystic phase of the dog tapeworm *Echinococcus* causes hydatid disease of man and sheep.

Schistosomiasis (*Schistosoma mansoni, S. japonicum*)

Distribution: countries requiring irrigation for agriculture

Lifecycle: adults exist in venous plexuses of the bowel wall, and produce eggs which are shed from the mucosa (some eggs enter the portal circulation and pass to the liver causing severe irritation and portal fibrosis); eggs develop in water and larvae invade snail (secondary host); infective larvae released in water and bore through human skin (causing swimmer's itch); young adults migrate to venous plexuses.

(*S. haematobium*)

Same lifecycle; inhabits venous plexus of bladder wall; associated with fibrosis, ureteric strictures, calcification and infection

Diagnosis: typical eggs of the schistosomes are visible in faeces or urine

Treatment: requires expertise; usually with niclosamide, oxamnaquine or praziquantel.

Drugs mentioned in this chapter

Drug	Indication	Usage and precautions
Ampicillin	Dysenteriae dysentery	Adult dose 250–500 mg 6-hourly orally; child's dose half of adult dose (amoxycillin has no advantage, as systemic absorption is not required)
Erythromycin	Severe or prolonged campylobacteriosis,	Adult dose 250–500 mg 6-hourly orally; child's dose half of adult dose
	For bacteraemias	Adult dose 300–500 mg 6-hourly by intravenous injection; child's dose 30–60 mg/kg daily in four doses
Mebendazole	Threadworms	All over 2 years: 100 mg single oral dose
	Roundworms, hookworms and whipworms	All over age 2 years: 100 mg 12-hourly orally for 3 days

Metronidazole	Amoebiasis and giardiasis	Adult dose 800 mg 8-hourly orally or 500 mg 8-hourly intravenously for 10–14 days; child's dose 7.5 mg/kg 8-hourly orally or by intravenous infusion
	Giardiasis only	Adult dose 2.0 g daily for 3 days
Piperazine	Threadworms and roundworms	Adult dose 4.0 g piperazine phosphate or hydrate with a purgative, e.g. senna tabs; the paralysed worms are passed in the faeces; a second dose is usually give 2 weeks later; child's dose is a third or two-thirds of adult dose
Streptomycin	Severe *sonnei* dysentery	Adult dose 1.0 g 6-hourly orally for 5 days; child's dose 250 mg 6-hourly; systemic toxicity is unlikely because the drug is not absorbed from the bowel
Tetracycline	Cholera	Usually oxytetracycline; adult dose 250–500 mg 6-hourly orally for 5 days; not usually available for children but justified in cholera; child's dose up to 2 years 62.5–125 mg daily in four divided doses; up to 5 years 250–500 mg daily in four divided doses; up to 12 years 500 mg–1.0 g daily in four divided doses; paediatric mixture 125 mg/5 ml is manufactured, and can be diluted
Thiabendazole	A toxic anthelmintic drug; treatment of choice for strongyloidiasis (also of use in toxocariasis and trichinosis)	Dose for all ages 25 mg/kg 12-hourly; in normal patients continued for 3 days; in immunosuppressed patients, or cases of hyperacute strongyloidiasis treatment may be continued for a month, and the dosage given 8-hourly for the first 3 days; gastrointestinal disturbance and allergic reactions are common (corticosteroids may help to alleviate these)

Trimethoprim	Flexner dysentery	Adult dose 200 mg 12-hourly orally; child's dose up to 6 months 25 mg 12-hourly orally; up to 5 years 50 mg 12-hourly orally; up to 12 years 100 mg 12-hourly orally
Vancomycin	Pseudomembranous colitis	Adult dose 125–500 mg 6-hourly orally; child's dose one-eighth to one half of adult dose; check blood levels, and try to use lowest effective dose, as sometimes absorption can occur through damaged bowel and ototoxicity could result

6

Enteric Fevers

Enteric fevers are different in many ways from the 'food poisoning' salmonella infections and to help in making the distinction they are included in this separate chapter. Firstly, while the thousands of food poisoning salmonellae are widely distributed in animals, birds and reptiles, *Salmonella typhi* and *S. paratyphi A, B* and *C* are found almost exclusively in man. Secondly, while food poisoning salmonellae are confined to the bowel, the enteric fever salmonellae cause a septicaemic illness and can affect any organ of the body. Thirdly, the food poisoning and enteric fever salmonellae are distinguishable from each other by cultural and biochemical differences seen in the laboratory.

Epidemiology
Transmission from man to man takes place by faecal–oral spread, often by consumption of water contaminated with the faeces of patients or asymptomatic carriers. The paratyphoid salmonellae may also be transmitted by food in which the organisms have multiplied after being introduced by a food handler, or by contaminated water. Shellfish may concentrate salmonellae introduced into estuaries with sewage, and are a recognized source of infection.

Paratyphoid fever can be contracted from milk and many diary products, including ice cream, but food hygiene laws in Britain go far to prevent this, by excluding carriers of the organisms from the food industry. *S. paratyphi B* has been isolated from birds and animals on occasions and these may be a rare source of infection.

In Britain, about 200 cases of typhoid fever and about 50 of paratyphoid A occur annually. The vast majority of these are imported from the Indian subcontinent. Most of the 50 or so cases of paratyphoid B are contracted in Europe and North Africa. About one-sixth of all enteric fevers appear to originate in Britain, but at least half of these cases are contacts of cases from abroad. Paratyphoid C is rarely reported.

Clinical features of typhoid fever
A brief attack of diarrhoea may quickly follow the ingestion of *S. typhi*. This is the 'illness of infection', and it is followed by an incubation period of 6–20 days, usually between 10 and 14 days. Typhoid fever begins with non-specific symptoms of which headache, dry cough, abdominal dis-

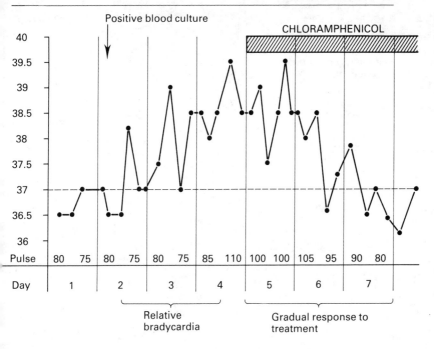

Fig. 13. Typical features in the chart of an enteric fever patient.

comfort and constipation are the most common. The temperature rises day by day in 'stepladder' fashion and, initially, the pulse is often not as elevated as expected for the degree of fever (Fig. 13). Some patients are confused and appear inattentive or deaf, while a few exhibit signs of severe paranoid psychosis, a diagnostic problem commonly encountered in some African endemic areas.

Usually by the second week the temperature has reached its height and the pulse has quickened. The spleen may be palpable and a variable rash may be seen. The rash consists of 2 mm diameter, hemispherical, pink spots ('rose spots') which blanch on pressure. A handful of spots may be scattered on the flanks or costal margins, or many may be present in various sites (Fig. 14). Diarrhoea due to inflammation of Peyer's patches now begins. It tends to be green and watery, often described as 'peasoup' stools. At this stage the patient is obviously ill and exhausted, and confusion or frank delirium may be expected.

By about the third week complications become a major problem. Although death may occur due to septicaemia and toxaemia in the early stages, complications are the commonest cause of death. They can occur even in treated patients.

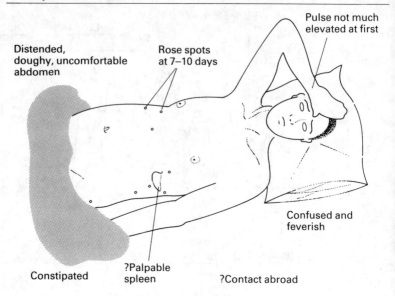

Pulse not much
elevated at first

Distended,
doughy, uncomfortable
abdomen

Rose spots
at 7–10 days

Confused and
feverish

Constipated

?Palpable
spleen

?Contact abroad

Fig. 14.   Early clinical signs of typhoid fever.

Bowel haemorrhage.   This is the commonest complication, occuring in up to 7 or 8% of patients. It results from erosion of Peyer's patches and varies from slight to life-threatening in degree.

Bowel perforation.   This usually occurs at the site of an ulcerated Peyer's patch. Some small perforations cause only local pain, tenderness and guarding, and may heal spontaneously; others result in generalized peritonitis.

Acute cholecystitis.   Although some inflammation of the gall bladder is usual in typoid fever, those patients with a tendency to acute cholecystitis may suffer an attack due to *S. typhi.*

Other manifestations.   Bronchitis, pneumonia, abscesses of kidney, skin or other organs, osteomyelitis and, rarely, meningitis may occur. Patients with sickle-cell disease are particularly susceptible to osteomyelitis.
   Children may be less severely affected by typhoid fever than adults. The absence of confusion, bradycardia or rose spots must not cause the physician to exclude the disease from the differential diagnosis of fever in a child. Small children and infants may suffer only a gastroenteritis-like illness.

Relapse. Up to 20% of patients who recover from untreated typhoid fever suffer a relapse, and this number can be doubled in inadequately treated cases. The relapse can vary from a few days' trivial illness to a recurrence of disease more severe than the original illness.

Clinical features of paratyphoid fever
The incubation period is shorter than that of typhoid fever, often in the region of a week and, although the course can be the same as that of typhoid fever, it more often takes the form of a severe, prolonged diarrhoeal illness. In general paratyphoid fever is a less severe and shorter illness than typhoid. Paratyphoid B is sometimes associated with a dense and widespread rash of rose spots.

Diagnosis
The white cell count is often rather low in enteric fever, due to an absolute neutropenia. Neutrophilia is sometimes seen in the earliest stages.

By cultures. During the 'illness of infection' stool cultures are transiently positive. The organism then passes into the lymphatic system, and its emergence into the blood marks the end of the incubation period. Blood cultures are usually positive for some days before the organism appears in the stool and are the most important diagnostic test. In some patients urine cultures also become positive.

The Widal test. In this test agglutinating antibody titres against H, O and Vi antigens are measured. The H antibody rises very early, and a titre of 64 or more in the unimmunized suggests active infection. A four-fold rise in O antibody is more likely to be detected in paired sera, as the H antibody titre is often already high at presentation; rising O antibody titres are therefore firm evidence of enteric fever. Vi antibodies are sometimes present in asymptomatic carriers. Although often quoted, the Widal test is a very poor diagnostic test in most cases because it is often confused by previous immunization or exposure.

Treatment
Because the mortality of untreated typhoid fever is up to 20% and because delay allows the development of serious complications, treatment should be commenced when there is reasonable evidence of the diagnosis, whether this is clinical, bacteriological or serological.

Most experts consider chloramphenicol to be the treatment of choice. This can be given orally unless the patient is too unwell to swallow it, in which case it must be given intravenously. Intravenous fluid and electrolyte replacement may be necessary in severely ill patients, and can be supplemented if needed with nutrients and vitamins. Chloramphenicol treatment is continued for 14 days. If a shorter course is given there is a high relapse rate; a longer course will not reduce the relapse rate below 5–10%. It is important to know that the temperature falls gradually to normal over a period of 3–5 days and clinical improvement cannot be expected before the second or third day of treatment, even when therapy is completely successful.

Some experienced clinicians find co-trimoxazole a useful drug for treatment of typhoid fever due to the strains of *S. typhi* found in the Indian subcontinent. It is given orally in high doses for about 2 weeks.

Ampicillin and amoxycillin sometimes appear to be effective, but are not reliably so.

Laboratory sensitivity tests may suggest that the organism is sensitive to several antibiotics but unfortunately do not reliably reflect the activity of the drug in the patient and should not, therefore, deter the clinician from using the treatment of choice. This means that chloramphenicol, or perhaps co-trimoxazole should be given unless there is a compelling contraindication.

Paratyphoid fever.   As with typhoid fever, *in vitro* sensitivity tests may be misleading. Chloramphenicol is the treatment of choice, though paratyphoid organisms sometimes prove resistant to it and are then extremely difficult to treat.

Side-effects of drugs.   Chloramphenicol is much feared as a cause of agranulocytosis. Although a drop of 10–20% in the white cell count often follows the commencement of chloramphenicol treatment, the incidence of further falls in the count is extremely low in patients with typhoid fever. The risk from chloramphenicol is considerably less than that from the disease. Co-trimoxazole less often causes blood dyscrasias, but the sulphonamide component is commonly responsible for skin reactions which are occasionally very severe.

Treatment of complications.   Metastatic infections will usually respond to the antibiotic therapy, and abscesses can be drained, if necessary, when the patient's condition has improved.

Bowel haemorrhage should be treated with whole-blood transfusion, supplemented in severe cases with fresh frozen plasma.

Bowel perforation is usually treated conservatively with gastric aspiration and intravenous fluid replacement. There is some evidence however that surgery can be of benefit in cases with generalized peritonitis, in spite of the friability of the gut and the extensive excision which is often required.

Follow-up
Medical Officers of Environmental Health usually require evidence of

three consecutive negative stool and early morning urine cultures before releasing a patient from surveillance. This number is increased to 12 negative stool cultures for some food handlers, water workers and nursery teachers. Specimens are examined twice weekly. Some patients are excretors of the organism for up to a year after recovery. If they excrete the organism after this they are regarded as carriers.

In the presence of gallstones carriage is likely to be permanent. Removal of the gallbladder then offers a 60–70% chance of clearance. Ampicillin is concentrated in the bile, and offers a chance of clearance if given in high doses for at least four weeks, but it is ineffective in the presence of gallstones.

Permanent carriers are excluded from the food industry. As long as their standard of personal hygiene is satisfactory they are not otherwise a significant public health hazard.

Prophylaxis
An inactivated vaccine against *S. typhi* is available. It is recommended to travellers intending to visit endemic areas.

An oral typhoid vaccine may become available in the near future.

Drugs mentioned in this chapter

Drug	Indication	Dosage and precautions
Chloramphenicol	Typhoid and paratyphoid fevers	Adult dose 500 mg 6-hourly orally or intravenously—patient over 70 kg may be given 1.0 g 8-hourly; child's dose 50–100 mg/kg daily in four divided doses *CAUTION*—neonates cannot metabolize chloramphenicol as quickly as adults; they may suffer accumulation, leading to the 'grey baby' syndrome; they may be given 25 mg/kg daily, with all care, if this is unavoidable; a few patients suffer an exacerbation of toxaemia when organisms are rapidly killed at the beginning of treatment. Halving the first dose may avoid this. Corticosteroids may ameliorate this reaction
Co-trimoxazole	Typhoid fever contracted in the Indian sub-continent; other-	Adult dose 1920 mg (4 × 480 mg tablets) twice-daily—patient under 70 kg may be given 3 × 480 mg tablets twice daily; dose

	wise the drug of second choice	may be reduced to 960 mg or 1440 mg (2 or 3 tablets) twice daily when the temperature has returned to normal; all doses are given orally; child's dose: 6 weeks to 5 months 180 mg twice daily; 6 months to 5 years 360 mg twice daily; 6–12 years 720 mg twice daily
Ampicillin or amoxycillin	Treatment of excreters or carriers with normally functioning gallbladders, or after cholecystectomy; not often successful in treating acute disease	Adult dose 500 mg to 1.0 g 6-hourly, orally for at least 4 weeks; child's dose 100 mg/kg daily in divided doses; duration of treatment may be reduced by a week or two if probenecid is given: adult dose 500 mg 6-hourly, child's dose 40 mg/kg daily

7

Hepatic Infections

The cells of the liver can be invaded by a variety of infectious agents which produce a feverish illness with liver cell damage. The most familiar agents of hepatitis are viruses, but a large number of others, including mycoplasmas, rickettsiae, protozoa and some bacteria can produce hepatitis as part of a more extensive illness. Hepatocellular disturbance is also common in septicaemia, though it is not known whether endotoxin or bacterial invasion is the cause.

Biliary infections usually result from infection of stagnant bile when the biliary tract is obstructed. The commonest cause of this is a gallstone, but malignant stricture is not unusual and fibrotic strictures can occur after surgery or other injury. The responsible micro-organisms are usually bacteria originating from the bowel, including both aerobic enterobacteriacae and anaerobes such as *Bacteroides spp.* and *Clostridium perfringens*. In the latter case, gas is formed and may outline the biliary tree in a plain abdominal X-ray. Biliary tract infection is one recognized precursor of acute pancreatitis.

Large-scale destruction of liver cells leads to abscess formation. This is a hazard of severe amoebic dysentery, but bacterial abscesses may also occur. These are often associated with other evidence of intra-abdominal sepsis, such as a perforated appendicitis or diverticulitis, or with a septicaemia, particularly staphylococcal septicaemia.

Symptoms and signs of liver infection

Jaundice. This is a usual finding in both obstructive liver disease, with or without biliary infection, and in hepatocellular disease. In both cases conjugated bilirubin is released into the bloodstream from the damaged liver and is excreted in the urine. The urine therefore looks dark or 'strong tea' coloured at an early stage. The stools are often pale due to failure of excretion of bile pigment.

It is difficult to distinguish clinically between obstructive (cholestatic, or posthepatic) and hepatocellular jaundice, though cholestasis is often associated with itching. Itching, however, can mark the onset and the convalescent phase of hepatitis, for cholestasis then occurs even though hepatocellular disorder predominates.

Pain. This may aid in distinction between hepatocellular or obstructive jaundice, as obstruction is commonly associated with biliary colic. A combination of right upper quadrant pain and a positive Murphy's sign (tenderness at the anterior end of the right ninth rib on inspiration) will suggest gall bladder inflammation, and may be reinforced by a history of previous similar episodes.

The pain associated with hepatitis is probably due to stretching of the liver capsule, and is diffuse and vague. It is often exacerbated by movement or by walking, and there is tenderness on palpation of the liver edge.

The pain of a liver abscess may be similar to that of hepatitis but is usually more severe. If the abscess is in the right lobe, local increased tenderness is often found over its site.

Caution: acholuric jaundice.   If no bile is present in the urine of a jaundiced patient, the jaundice is probably due to unconjugated bilirubinaemia resulting from haemolysis. Haemolysis occurs in sickle-cell disease, glucose-6-phosphate dehydrogenase deficiency, malaria, some mycoplasma infections and some septicaemias. It is unwise, therefore, to make a diagnosis of hepatitis in the absence of bilirubinuria.

Non-infectious causes of jaundice.   These are manifold and must be considered, if only to be excluded, before a diagnosis of infection is made. Important causes are: biliary obstruction without infection, drug reactions or toxicity, alcoholic hepatitis, collagen and autoimmune diseases, malignant infiltration and haemolysis due to red blood cell disorders, drug reactions, autoimmune disease or malignancy.

Investigation of infective jaundice
Urinary urobilinogen.   This is elevated above the upper limit of normal in the early and the recovery phase of infective hepatitis. The reason for this is not known but, paradoxically, the raised urobilinogen often coincides with episodes of mild cholestasis. In obstructive jaundice, urobilinogen levels are low or undetectable.

Aspartate transaminase (AST, SGOT).   This enzyme originates from liver, muscle and brain cells. It reaches high levels in the blood during the onset of hepatitis. Exact levels are very variable, but peaks of 1000–2000 i.u./l are not unusual. Levels of 3000 i.u./l or more indicate very severe damage. Alanine transaminase (ALT, SGPT) is a specific liver cell transaminase.

Alkaline phosphatase.   This enzyme is elaborated by the cells lining the gallbladder and biliary tree. It may rise to three or four times its normal upper limit during hepatitis, but is much more elevated in cholestatic conditions and in biliary obstruction. Gamma-glutamyl transpeptidase

(γGT), is also a sensitive indicator of cholestasis, but is too easily altered by trivial conditions to be much used in the diagnosis of infection.

Caution. Children have high levels of alkaline phosphatase originating from growing bone (5'-nucleotidase is a specific liver phosphatase).

Blood glucose. Most of the glucose in the blood is derived from breakdown of liver glycogen. In severe hepatocellular disorder the blood glucose level can quickly fall to near zero.

Blood urea. Blood urea is manufactured from ammonia in the liver. Liver failure is associated with blood ureas much below the normal lower limit of about 2 mmol/l.

Clotting factors. Clotting factors have a very fast rate of destruction, and in liver failure they are not replaced. A much prolonged prothrombin time (PT) or partial thromboplastin time (PTT) gives early warning of potentially severe liver failure.

Ultrasound scan. This is a useful, non-invasive technique which, in experienced hands, can demonstrate gallstones, dilated bile ducts and parenchymal lesions such as abscesses. It is able to confirm a presumed diagnosis in a majority of such cases. In hepatitis there is no typical ultrasound finding but a confusion of signals from oedematous areas often produces a picture known as 'a bright liver'.

Isotope scans. In standard technetium scans, liver abscesses of 2 cm diameter or more can be seen as 'cold areas'.

Biopsy. This is rarely indicated in infection, but may demonstrate typical histology in some conditions such as acute infectious hepatitis, yellow fever and systemic leishmaniasis. *Aspiration of abscesses* can be of value in making a bacteriological diagnosis and as an aid to healing. It may be carried out under ultrasound control.

Serology. This is important. The accurate diagnosis of various types of hepatitis depends on the detection of specific antigens or antibodies in the serum. In some cases serological findings are related to the long-term prognosis.

Viral hepatitis

Many viruses may be associated with hepatitis syndromes, the initial clinical features of which are very similar to each other. The different viral syndromes can be distinguished by epidemiological and serological characteristics, and by their differing long-term effects. Three main viral syndromes are recognized: hepatitis A, hepatitis B and non-A–non-B hepatitis. These will be considered as the differential diagnosis of viral hepatitis.

Epidemiology of hepatitis A (infectious hepatitis)
This is a worldwide infection which spreads mainly by direct faecal–oral transfer in children, or in adults by ingestion of water contaminated by infected faeces, particularly in tropical countries. Shellfish may concentrate the virus from their contaminated surroundings, and are a recognized source of infection. Some outbreaks appear to have resulted from urinary contamination of food.

The incubation period is 2–6 weeks, usually 3–4. Patients excrete virus in their faeces for 1 or 2 weeks before and after the appearance of symptoms.

Epidemiology of hepatitis B (serum hepatitis)
This infection is spread by the parenteral route. Recognized risk factors are inoculation in blood transfusion, haemodialysis, shared intravenous needles, tattooing, ear piercing, acupunture, sexual contact or bites from infected persons. The infection is particularly common in renal dialysis patients, intravenous drug abusers and homosexual men. It is sometimes present in mentally retarded people who reside in institutions.

The incubation period is from 3 to 6 months, and virus, or virus fragments are excreted in the urine, faeces, saliva and semen from a few weeks before the onset of symptoms for up to 3 months after illness. Patients with tolerance due to repeated exposure, or with altered immunity may 'carry' virus or virus fragments in the blood for an indefinite period.

Infants born to certain carrier mothers or to women suffering from hepatitis B are likely to become permanent carriers, probably following mild infection. In some parts of the world, particularly Indonesian and some Asian regions this 'vertical transmission' increases the carrier rate to 15 or 20%. In Northern Europe and America the average number of carriers is about one in 500–1000 people.

Epidemiology of non-A–non-B hepatitis
This is currently being studied. It is likely that there are two main categories of non-A–non-B hepatitis; that with an incubation period of 1–3 weeks which commonly follows transfusion of blood products, and that with an incubation period of 6–10 weeks which occurs in patients who have travelled abroad, as well as in transfused patients.

Among British and American populations, up to 11% of hepatitis cases are not due to hepatitis A, hepatitis B or a variety of other agents, and are classed as non-A–non-B.

Clinical features of viral hepatitis

A prodromal illness of 2–7 days occurs, with exhaustion, anorexia, nausea and sometimes vomiting. It is said to be longer, with some arthralgia and occasionally a faint rash in hepatitis B, but this is rarely clinically important and does not allow distinction of hepatitis B from other types on clinical grounds. The prodromal illness of hepatitis A is sometimes accompanied by a high, swinging fever.

The onset of jaundice is indicated by the darkening of the urine and lightening of the stools. There is often tenderness and slight enlargement of the liver. The jaundice is rarely accompanied by fever. It lasts usually from 1 to 3 weeks, but is occasionally prolonged. In hepatitis A jaundice of of 6–12 months' duration sometimes occurs, often associated with mild cholestasis and pruritis, but recovery is eventually complete. In hepatitis B a few patients have lifelong serological evidence of persisting viral infection, and a few of these continue to have liver inflammation (chronic active hepatitis). They may develop antinuclear and smooth muscle antibodies, and some cases progress to cirrhosis and eventual liver failure.

Children in particular may have a mild or non-icteric course, the only indication of illness being a little vomiting, a few loose stools or transiently darkened urine. Bile is often detectable on 'stick testing' of the urine and plasma transaminases may be slightly elevated. These children easily pass infection to their attendants and playmates.

Complications

Liver failure. This may occur so early in the course of the illness that jaundice never develops, or it may progress inexorably over a period of 1 or more weeks. About one-third of affected patients have serological evidence of hepatitis B. The patient often vomits on several occasions and becomes uncooperative and drowsy. Constructional apraxia (inability to copy a sketch of a five-pointed star, but relative ease in drawing a square) is a useful early sign. Eventually the patient becomes comatose.

Initially the transaminase levels are very high, but they fall as the liver is destroyed. The blood glucose and blood urea are low, clotting factors are depleted, and death from hypoglycaemia, intoxication with accumulating amines or haemorrhage soon follows.

There are typical slow waves in the electroencephalograph of patients with hepatic coma.

Aplastic anaemia. This is a rare but serious complication of non-B hepatitis. It usually occurs during the convalescent phase, and is profound and irreversible. The best hope of cure is through bone marrow transplantation, so blood transfusions should be kept to a minimum to avoid antibody formation, and specialist advice should be sought early.

Diagnosis
The white cell count tends to be low in viral hepatitis, due to mild neutropenia. Neutrophilia may occur in acute hepatic necrosis.

Hepatitis A. Diagnosis is confirmed by the presence of IgM-class antibodies to hepatitis A virus (antiHAV-IgM) in the serum; (antiHAV-IgG indicates past infection, and is detectable in 50% or more of various adult populations).

Hepatitis B (Fig. 15). Three substances are detectable in the serum before the onset of clinical illness and raised serum transaminases. The first to appear, 2–8 weeks before illness, is the *hepatitis B surface antigen* (HBsAg), formerly called Australia antigen and probably representing a surface fragment of hepatitis B virus. Just before the illness the *e antigen* (HBeAg) appears, accompanied by *DNA polymerase*. These are markers of replicating virus. They are associated with high infectivity and the presence of whole virus particles in the blood.

As illness begins, *core antibody* (antiHBc) appears, although free HBcAg is not seen. This antibody is an indicator of infection, which persists long after the illness is over. *AntiHBe* appears soon after *antiHBc* and is associated with gradual clearance of HBeAg and reduction of infectivity.

Late in convalescence, *antiHBs* appears.

In some patients HBsAg persists indefinitely in the serum, and a few of these patients also have persisting HBeAg. Those with HBeAg are more infectious, more likely to have progressive liver disease and, if pregnant, are more likely to infect their newborn children.

The usual diagnostic test for hepatitis B is the detection of HBsAg in the serum. The other serological changes help to distinguish cases from long-term carriers.

Non-A–non-B hepatitis. At present there is no specific diagnostic test for this group. Exclusion of common viral infections such as hepatitis A, hepatitis B, infectious mononucleosis and cytomegalovirus allows a probable diagnosis to be made.

Treatment of viral hepatitis
There is no specific treatment for the viral infection. Bedrest is helpful in reducing malaise, and there is some evidence that ambulation while the transaminases are elevated to more than five times the normal upper limit can delay recovery. Patients usually feel most ill before the jaundice appears. After the appetite returns the patient may take what diet he pleases; restriction of fat intake does not seem to offer any advantage.

A few patients with cholestasis are sometimes helped symptomatically by small doses of antihistamines, which ameliorate pruritus.

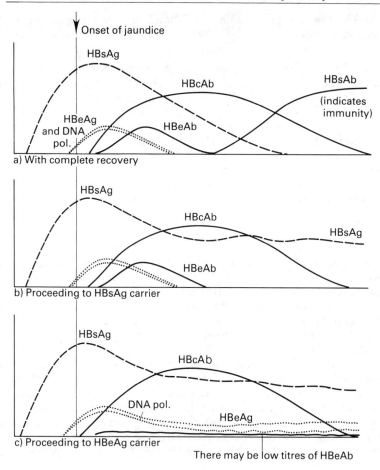

Fig. 15. Antigens and antibodies in the diagnosis of hepatitis B.

Prolonged jaundice. When bilirubinuria and elevation of transaminases persist for more than 6 weeks in hepatitis A, there is often evidence of cholestasis. Severe pruritis is accompanied by alkaline phosphatase levels of four or five times normal. In this situation it is often helpful to administer prednisolone 30–40 mg daily. The cholestasis is relieved and jaundice improves in about 1 week, after which the prednisolone dosage can be gradually reduced.

Prolonged jaundice in hepatitis B may indicate the presence of chronic liver disease. Persistence of HBeAg and DNA polymerase will indicate the likelihood of progression to cirrhosis, as will the appearance of autoantibodies.

Liver failure.   This is a serious problem for which modern medicine, including pig liver perfusion, haemodialysis and charcoal perfusion, has no easy remedy. Treatment is based on vigorous supportive measures to allow time for natural recovery. Plentiful intravenous glucose should be given to correct hypoglycaemia. The elaboration of amines by bowel organisms should be minimized by giving a low-protein diet, by purging with magnesium sulphate or lactulose and by administration of oral neomycin. Clotting factors should be replaced with fresh blood or fresh frozen plasma infusions whenever haemorrhage threatens. In many units cimetidine or ranitidine is given to reduce the likelihood of bleeding from acute gastric erosions.

Prevention of viral hepatitis

The acquisition of hepatitis A is avoided by the use of safe, or boiled, water for drinking and food preparation, and by adherence to strict standards of personal hygiene, particularly to washing the hands frequently.

Hepatitis B is controlled by surveillance and exclusion of infected blood products and by single use of disposable intravenous cannulae in hospitals. HBsAg-positive patients are segregated from others in renal dialysis units.

Normal human immunoglobulin (HIG) contains antibodies to hepatitis A, and will provide short-term protection for travellers to endemic areas. Hepatitis B immune globulin (HBIG) is given immediately after exposure to infection (never later than 48 hours afterwards) and again 1 month later to protect against the longer-incubation hepatitis B. It can also be useful in the prophylactic treatment of infants born to infected, or HBeAg-positive mothers, though more than one monthly booster is usually required in these cases.

Active immunization against hepatitis B has recently become available. The inactivated vaccine is recommended for some high-risk groups, and may be useful in the future for post-exposure prophylaxis.

Yellow fever

Epidemiology

This is a viraemic disease due to a group B arbovirus. It is transmitted from monkeys to man (sylvatic cycle) in tropical forests, and from man to man (urban cycle) by *Aedes spp.* mosquitoes. It occurs widely in central Africa, central and south America and parts of the Caribbean, but the immunization of travellers under the International Health Regulations normally prevents its entry into non-endemic areas.

Clinical features
After 3–6 days incubation period, illness begins abruptly with headache, myalgia, conjuctival redness, high fever, nausea and vomiting. Bradycardia is common. A furred tongue with a bright red border is characteristic. After about 3 days the temperature falls, but in severe cases it rises again and the pulse remains slow. Jaundice then appears, but is less prominent than the severe bleeding manifestations, of which 'black vomit' is the most sinister. Coma may follow, with a brief excitable period just before death.

In mild cases there may be no second fever, perhaps only albuminuria or epistaxis, while in fulminant cases there may be no interval between the two feverish phases.

Diagnosis
A low white cell count with neutropenia is usual in the first week of illness. The virus can be isolated from the blood, or rising antibody titres detected in paired sera. The liver shows characteristic histological features with acidophilic, necrotic *Councilman bodies*.

Specimens from suspected yellow fever patients should be sent only to specially designated laboratories (see Chapter 20).

Treatment and prevention
There is no specific treatment but, with supportive therapy, the mortality rate is often less than 10%.

Effective immunization is available with a live attenuated group D arbovirus. Immunization is required for travellers to endemic areas, in accordance with International Health Regulations.

Leptospirosis

Epidemiology
Leptospirosis is a zoonosis, a disease acquired from animals which hardly ever passes from man to man. Different types of leptospira are excreted in the urine of various animals. *Leptospira icterohaemorrhagiae* is present in the urine of rats, *L. canicola* in the urine of dogs and *L. pomona*, *L. hebdomadis*, *L. autumnalis* and others in the urine of various rodents or, sometimes, pigs.

Man usually becomes infected by contact of contaminated water with skin lesions or mucosal surfaces. Sewer workers, miners, fish farm workers, canal holidaymakers, builders and farmers are among those most affected. Direct contact with infected animals or carcasses may also lead to infection.

Clinical features
Leptospira icterohaemorrhagiae is capable of producing Weil's disease,

the most serious form of leptospirosis. After an incubation period of 2–4 weeks the patient develops high fever, headache and myalgia. The majority of patients have hepatocellular jaundice and conjuctival inflammation. Up to half have signs of meningitis. A minority of patients develop a rash which may be petechial or haemorrhagic, though serious bleeding problems are rare. There is usually biochemical evidence of renal impairment.

L. canicola is associated with canicola fever, a milder disease than Weil's disease, often only consisting of febrile or meningeal manifestations. Mild influenza-like illness with headache and myalgia is common in all types of infection. This is self-limiting and rarely lasts longer than 1 week.

Diagnosis
There is often a moderate neutrophil leukocytosis. In cases with meningitis an excess of lymphocytes is found in the cerebrospinal fluid (CSF), and CSF protein is slightly raised. There is usually albuminuria.

Leptospira can be isolated from blood, and sometimes CSF, in the first few days of illness. They may also be demonstrated in urine, blood or CSF by dark-ground microscopy or special silver-stained preparations.

Serological examination of paired sera is the most common method of diagnosis. This is best carried out in a reference laboratory, as experience is necessary to interpret the various cross-reactions between groups of leptospira.

Treatment
The mild forms rarely require specific treatment. Severe illness with jaundice, meningitis, bleeding or renal impairment is usually treated with intravenous benzylpenicillin. Tetracycline has been suggested if penicillin is contraindicated. Chloramphenicol is known to be ineffective.

Prevention
Control of rats and other rodents is important in agricultural and industrial areas. Avoidance of contact with river, canal and pond water is advisable.

Immunization against Weil's disease is available for those who risk heavy exposure, for example sewerage workers.

Cholecystitis

Epidemiology
This infection is usually associated with gallstones or other obstructive abnormalities of the biliary tree, which predispose to stagnation of bile and subsequent bacterial invasion. The organisms responsible for invasion are bowel organisms, including *Escherichia coli* and other Enterobacteriacae, *Bacteroides spp.* and *Clostridium perfringens*.

Clinical features
Fever is associated with right hypochondrial pain and a positive Murphy's sign. There may be pale stools, dark urine, frank jaundice and pruritis. There is often a history of previous mild attacks, of pain following fat ingestion or of known gallstones.

Diagnosis
Liver function tests reveal a typical pattern of cholestasis. Only 15% of gallstones are visible on the plain abdominal X-ray. Ultrasound scanning may demonstrate dilated bile ducts or gallstones. Oral cholecystography and intravenous cholangiography are only possible when there is little or no jaundice.

Blood cultures are positive in some cases.

Treatment
Intravenous fluid administration, analgesics and antibiotics are usually given. Ampicillin is concentrated in the bile, and is a good first choice of antibiotic. If there is no response to ampicillin, gentamicin and metronidazole may be given.

If blood cultures are positive, identification and sensitivity testing will aid the choice of antibiotic.

Elective surgical intervention is often indicated.

Liver abscess

Epidemiology
Bacterial liver abscesses are usually associated with intra-abdominal sepses, such as appendicitis or diverticulitis, or with bowel surgery. In this case they are usually due to bowel organisms, often faecal streptococci or anaerobic organisms.

Occasionally liver abscess complicates a septicaemia, and may then be due to staphylococci, salmonellae or other unusual organisms.

Clinical features
Swinging fever, tender enlargement of the liver and neutrophil leukocytosis are the usual features. Adjacent pleural effusion or lung atelectasis may be present. The development of liver abscess may be difficult to distinguish from coexisting intra-abdominal sepsis, and many abscesses are undiagnosed in life.

Diagnosis
A large abscess or abscesses may be delineated by ultrasound, isotope or computed tomographic scanning. Multiple small abscesses may be undetectable.

Positive cultures may be obtained from needle aspirate of an abscess or from blood cultures.

Treatment
This may have to be 'blind', in which case a combination of metronidazole with gentamicin, cefotaxime, ampicillin, mezlocillin or
azlocillin is advisable. Otherwise antibiotic choice is dictated by the
results of cultures. Drainage by needle aspiration or open surgery is
carried out, if feasible.

Subphrenic abscess

This problem often results in prolonged fever and toxaemia after
abdominal trauma or surgery. The features are similar to those of liver
abscess, except that signs in the adjacent lung and pleura are almost
always present.

The crescent-shaped abscess may defy detection by fluoroscopic screening of diaphragmatic movement and by all other available imaging techniques, only to be revealed by exploratory needling or surgery. Clinical
suspicion is therefore important in making the diagnosis.

Surgical drainage is mandatory. Antibiotic therapy is also important,
and should be based on the results of pus or blood cultures if possible.

Drugs mentioned in this chapter

Drug	Indication	Dosage and precautions
Benzylpenicillin	Leptospirosis	Adult dose 1.2–2.4 g (2–4 mega units) 6-hourly, intravenously; child's dose is a quarter to half of adult dose
Ampicillin or amoxycillin	Cholecystitis	Adult dose 1.0 g 6-hourly; child's dose is a quarter to half of adult dose
Gentamicin cefotaxime mezlocillin }	Wide-spectrum anti-Gram-negative agents	For treatment of hepatic and subphrenic abscess; for doses, see Chapter 10, page 136
Azlocillin	Wide-spectrum, may be used if *Pseudomonas* is causing disease and renal problems exclude use of aminoglycosides	
Metronidazole	For infection with anaerobic organisms	

8

Urinary Tract Infections

Introduction
For the purpose of describing infectious processes, the urinary tract can conveniently be considered in three parts: the urethra, the bladder, and the kidneys and ureters.

The urethra
In both men and women, the urethra is closely associated with the genital tract, in men because it provides a pathway from the vas deferens to the exterior, and in women because it is continuous with the vulva. In contrast with the rest of the urinary tract, which is lined with transitional epithelium, the main lining of the urethra is of columnar epithelium, with stratified squamous epithelium at its meatus.

Sexually transmissible diseases can affect both male and female urethra. Infections arising elsewhere in the urinary tract are often associated with urethritis, and the urethra is also considered to be a means of entry for ascending urinary tract infection. In some women, the same organism may be isolated from the urine, the perineum, the vulva and the vagina.

Abnormalities of the urethra. These can dispose the urethra and the urinary tract to infection. The commonest abnormality is the presence of strictures or congenital valves, which encourage retention and stasis of urine. A urethral catheter constitutes a foreign body which is likely to produce a tissue reaction, and which prevents the normal cleansing action of urine flow over the mucosa.

The bladder
This can be affected by ascending infection via the urethra, or sometimes by infection progressing downwards from the kidneys. It has been suggested that bacteria able to adhere to the transitional epithelium, by means of pili or fimbriae, are more likely to be pathogenic in the urinary tract. Certain strains of *Escherichia coli* are known to have this adhesive property, and the degree to which they adhere to mucosa varies from person to person, perhaps depending on genetic predisposition.

Abnormalities of the bladder.   The bladder sphincter affords a protective seal against the influx of infection from the urethra. A faulty sphincter, as in mechanical disorder or neuromuscular disease, predisposes the patient to bladder infection. Holding the sphincter open with a catheter has similar effects.

The existence of diverticula or of obstruction to bladder outflow by an enlarged prostate, a tumour or stone, all contribute to retention and stagnation of urine with subsequent infection. A stone, tumour or foreign body in the bladder may also provide a source of infection which will only be eradicated by removal of the cause, even though antibiotic treatment may provide temporary relief.

The kidneys and ureters

These constitute the upper urinary tract. Infection here can arise by extension from the bladder, particularly if there is vesicoureteric reflux. This occurs in some children, in the lax urinary tract of pregnant women, and in the presence of back-pressure from an obstructed bladder outflow. Stones, tumours or strictures obstructing the renal pelvis or ureters can give rise to infection in stagnant urine. Extension of infection into the pyramids and tubules of the kidneys of small children can lead to chronic pyelonephritis and parenchymal kidney damage.

The rich blood supply of the kidney can bring infection via the bloodstream in bacteraemic or septicaemic states. This often results in abscess formation, and such organisms as *Staphylococcus aureus*, coliform bacilli, salmonellae and anaerobes may then be excreted in the urine.

Symptoms and signs

Frequency of micturition.   This is usually due to irritation of the trigone of the bladder or of the urethra. It occurs in urethritis and cystitis, and is the commonest symptom in these disorders.

Caution.   Frequency of micturition is not necessarily due to infection. Excess urine production will also cause it. This occurs in diabetes mellitus and in some types of renal failure, as well as in rarer conditions such as diabetes insipidus and drug reactions. Mechanical disorder of the bladder neck occurs in pregnancy and in some pelvic conditions, resulting in quite marked frequency, which is sometimes associated with infection.

Urgency of micturition.   This, an immediate necessity to micturate, is due to the same causes as frequency. In some cases it is so severe as to result in *urge incontinence* before the patient can take appropriate action. In the aged and the very young, incontinence is often regarded as inevitable, but many cases are probably due to infection, and could be alleviated by simple treatment.

Caution. Urgency of micturition can occur in several non-infectious conditions including prostatism, haematuria, passage of a stone or 'sand' and chemical irritation of the bladder or urethra.

Dysuria. This is painful micturition. In infection it is often an unpleasant burning sensation in the perineum and urethra, and it lasts for a short time during and after micturition. It is sometimes accompanied by suprapubic aching or burning. It can occur in both infectious and non-infectious conditions.

Renal pain. This is a poorly localized, aching pain which is felt in the small of the back, or high on the affected side. It can be sufficiently distressing to cause vomiting, which is quite a common occurrence in upper urinary tract infections. Palpation of the back, in the angle between the ribs and the spine, or ballotting the kidney between the anterior and posterior abdominal walls, may elicit tenderness and guarding on the affected side. Renal pain can occur in kidney infections without accompanying frequency, urgency or dysuria.

Non-specific signs and symptoms. These are common. They include nausea, meningism, diarrhoea and rigors, the latter being seen in cases of pyelonephritis, particularly those with bacteraemia. These signs can be useful indicators when more direct evidence of urinary tract infection is lacking.

Urinary signs. The patient may notice that the urine smells fishy or sharp. This is due to the ammonia and amines produced by the action of bacterial urease on urinary urea. Infected urine is often cloudy because of the presence of pus cells, and in severe infections sufficient red blood cells may be present to colour the urine pink or red.

Laboratory tests
Observation: the 'three-glass test'. In this test, the urine is passed, in approximately equal volume, into three glass containers. The initial container will contain urine with urethral contents, the second container collects a midstream specimen (presumed to be bladder urine) and the last, in men, contains the terminal urine with any prostatic secretions. The specimens are examined for threads of mucin which can be seen in the first glass if urethritis is present, and in the last if prostatitis exists.

Side-ward tests. Simple tests can be used to determine the pH of urine and its chemical constituents. In ammonia-producing infection the urinary pH can be high, in the region of 8 or 9, while 'normal' urine usually has a pH of 4–6. The presence of protein or blood in the sample will also indicate an abnormality of the urinary tract, which may be an infection.

Examination of the midstream urine sample (MSU).   This is considered to be a sample of bladder urine, which is normally sterile. Direct light microscopy of the urine will reveal the presence of pus cells (neutrophil leukocytes), which indicates a likelihood of infection. Pus cells are not seen in normal urine. Urine sediment may be Gram-stained, and organisms such as coliforms or gonococci can usefully be sought in this way.

Quantitative culture is carried out by using a standard sized silver loop to 'plate out' cultures. The presence of more than 10^8 colony-forming units per litre (more than 10^5/ml organisms) is traditionally taken to indicate true infection while less organisms may indicate only contamination of the specimen. In practice, symptomatic infections with pus cells visible in the MSU are sometimes associated with a low number of organisms detectable. Treatment should not be withheld because of this. Causes of low bacterial counts include polyuria, frequent bladder emptying, recent antibiotic therapy and contamination of the specimen with disinfectant. In addition, some fastidious organisms such as anaerobes, chlamydiae and mycoplasmas can be difficult to culture.

'Sterile pyuria' (abacterial pyuria).   This is the term applied to those cases where repeated urine samples show pus cells, but fail to produce bacterial growth. Urinary symptoms may or may not be present. The causes of low bacterial counts may also cause sterile pyuria. Infection with chlamydiae or with mycoplasmas is probably quite a common cause. Other infectious causes include genitourinary tuberculosis, brucellosis, and abdominal infection adjacent to the urinary tract (for instance appendicitis or diverticular abscess).

Mechanical causes such as stone or tumour can produce sterile pyuria, and chemical cystitis is associated with the use of certain drugs, particularly cyclophosphamide.

Asymptomatic bacteriuria (covert bacteriuria).   Screening tests in population groups shows that 2–5% of girls and women, and about one-tenth this proportion of boys and men, excrete significant numbers of bacteria in the urine. This is a fluctuating situation in which many people stop excreting bacteria, while others begin, all the time.

In normal adults, asymptomatic bacteriuria is probably benign. In children aged less than 4 years, however, the risk of chronic pyelonephritis following urinary infection is relatively high and all bacteriuria should probably be treated. In pregnancy, bacteriuria rarely disappears spontaneously and often leads to symptomatic infection. Those with diabetes or prostatism may also require treatment if bacteriuria is discovered.

Suprapubic aspiration of urine. This is a valuable investigation in babies and in others who are unable to provide specimens such as midstream urine samples upon request. The distended bladder is aspirated via a cannula, passed under aseptic conditions, into the extraperitoneal part of the bladder just above the pubic symphysis. Normally such bladder urine is sterile, so that the presence of any organisms, with or without pus cells, can be taken to indicate infection.

Imaging studies. Intravenous urography (IVU) or intravenous pyelography (IVP) is valuable in detecting abnormalities of all parts of the urinary tract. It will demonstrate obstruction to flow, vesicoureteric reflux, tumours, diverticula, distortion of the calyces of the renal pelvis, scarring of the renal parenchyma and congenital abnormalities of the renal tract.

Recurrent urinary tract infection is a strong indication for IVU examination.

Ultrasound scanning of the kidneys is useful in detecting cysts, which may appear similar to solid lesions on IVU. Aspiration of cyst contents can be carried out under ultrasound control.

Urethritis and 'the urethral syndrome'

Epidemiology
This condition, of inflammation of the urethra, is common and comes to the attention of general physicians and specialists in sexually transmitted diseases as often as to that of the infectious diseases specialist. In men particularly, urethritis is a feature of gonorrhoea and of non-specific sexually transmitted diseases as well as of urinary tract infection.

'Non-specific' organisms affecting both sexes include *Chlamydia trachomatis*, *Mycoplasma hominis* and *Ureaplasma urealyticum*. Urinary tract pathogens often seen include *Escherichia coli*, *Proteus spp.* and faecal streptococci which are probably derived from the bowel flora, either ascending from the perineum or descending from the infected bladder. Organisms previously thought to be of no significance, such as *Staphylococcus saprophyticus* are increasingly recognized as pathogenic in the urinary tract, and, although factors such as tight clothing or irritating soaps and perfumes probably play a part in the aetiology of urethritis, the disorder is nowadays more likely to be considered infectious than otherwise.

Some women have recurrent attacks of urethritis, often related to sexual intercourse. Evidence of infection may be lacking and the illness is then known as the 'urethral syndrome'.

Clinical features
A typical feature is urgency of micturition, which often results in frequency and may cause the need to void urine every 15–30 minutes. Pain

on micturition is often described as burning and, in men, a urethral discharge may be noticed, particularly before the first morning urine is passed. Local reddening sometimes occurs at the urethral meatus.

Fever, leukocytosis and lymph node swelling are rarely noticeable.

Diagnosis
It is advisable in some cases to take urethral swabs in order to exclude gonococcal infection. Immediate microscopy in this case will often reveal many pus cells together with intracellular and extracellular Gram-negative diplococci. The results of culture will confirm the diagnosis. Swabs may be taken into special media for the identification of chlamydiae in tissue culture. In the majority of cases the MSU reveals the presence of pus cells and small numbers of bacteria. These should not be dismissed as contaminants, for research has shown that they are often associated with the presence of bacteria in suprapubic bladder aspirates, and therefore signify a true infection.

If no organism can be detected by these means, it is still possible that a mycoplasma or ureaplasma is involved, though few laboratories offer routine cultural facilities for these. The genitalia should be examined for evidence of herpes simplex and swabs should be taken for the detection of *Candida albicans* or *Trichomonas vaginalis*, as these can cause vulvitis and urethral irritation in women, and balanitis with urethritis in men.

In those patients who have persistent or recurrent urethritis without detectable pathogens, sparse pus cells can often be found on urethral swabbing.

Treatment
More than half of cases, those with bacteria detectable in MSU culture, will respond to treatment with antibiotics. The antibiotic of choice will depend ultimately on the results of sensitivity testing, but success is likely with trimethoprim, co-trimoxazole and sometimes ampicillin or amoxycillin. *Staph. saprophyticus* infection should be treated with flucloxacillin. All of these drugs are concentrated in the urine, and adequate local concentrations of antibiotic can be achieved with oral administration.

Chlamydial and other 'non-specific' infections will usually respond to treatment with tetracycline or erythromycin, given orally. A 2–3 weeks course is often required for complete cure.

The usual treatment for gonorrhea is a single dose of 3 g ampicillin given orally with probenecid. Daily intramuscular procaine penicillin with probenecid for 14–21 days is also used as it is effective against syphilis as well. An increasing number of gonococci are becoming resistant to penicillin; intramuscular cefuroxime or spectinomycin is given in this case.

Sufferers from the urethral syndrome are rarely helped by antibiotic treatment. Measures such as drinking a tumbler of fluid before retiring, and voiding urine after intercourse are sometimes very helpful in reducing the number and severity of episodes.

Caution. Urgency of micturition in middle-aged and elderly men is a common feature of prostatism. Rectal examination will reveal the enlarged prostate gland.

In women of a similar age-group, urethral caruncle is common. This is a pea-sized, pedunculated, vascular mass which arises from the posterior urethral wall near the meatus. It is always associated with urethritis, and may bleed after micturition. Surgical removal is required.

Cystitis

Epidemiology
This is a very common infection which is thought to result most often from microbial invasion of the bladder via the urethra. About half of all adult women suffer from at least one attack of cystitis during their lives and infection is also seen, though less commonly, in children and in adult men. The contribution of outflow obstruction and of foreign bodies has already been discussed. In particular, enlargement of the prostate is often associated with cystitis in elderly men.

The most common pathogen is *E. coli*; less common are *Proteus spp.*, other Gram-negative bacilli, faecal streptococci and *Staph. saprophyticus*. In patients who have predisposition to bladder infection, wide-spectrum antibiotic therapy may be followed by invasion with antibiotic-resistant klebsiellae or *Pseudomonas spp.*

Clinical features
These include frequency and urgency of micturition, burning dysuria and distressing suprapubic discomfort. Fever is common, but is not always present.

The patient may notice that the urine is cloudy or bloodstained and that it has an offensive smell. Infection with urease-producing organisms such as *Proteus* spp. is associated with production of ammonia, which has a characteristic smell, and which causes exacerbations of nappy rash in babies.

Diagnosis
Ward testing of the urine often shows the presence of protein or blood. The patient's blood film usually, but not always, demonstrates a neutrophil leukocytosis.

Firm diagnosis rests on finding a significant number of bacteria ($10^8/1$ or more), with pus cells, in the midstream urine specimen (MSU). In the presence of typical symptoms and pus cells in the urine, however, a finding of less than $10^8/1$ bacteria may be considered diagnostic.

Treatment
Escherichia coli is by far the most common infecting agent, and outside hospital it is often sensitive to ampicillin or amoxycillin. Sulphonamides such as sulphamethizole and sulphafurazole are also effective and are less likely to produce severe side-effects than the long-acting sulphonamides.

The optimum duration of treatment in uncomplicated infections is controversial. It is likely that 2 or 3 days is quite long enough, and indeed some workers have given just one or two large doses of ampicillin, with satisfactory results. The more conventional approach is to give 7–10 days of treatment.

Hospital-acquired infections and resistant community-acquired infections may respond to treatment with trimethoprim. Trimethoprim combined with sulphonamide (co-trimoxazole) is effective in more than three-quarters of cases of cystitis and has the advantage that the two components prevent the development of resistance to one another. The long-acting sulphonamide component, however, can cause rashes and feverish reactions.

Urinary antimicrobial drugs which have very low blood levels, but adequate urine levels, are sometimes useful when it is desirable to avoid the systemic effects of antibiotics. Nitrofurantoin has a fairly wide spectrum of activity against Gram-negative bacteria in the urine, and nalidixic acid is also of some use, though its spectrum is narrower.

Infections with highly resistant organisms may require treatment with wide-spectrum cephalosporins, penicillins or aminoglycosides. If such treatment is contemplated, it is usually for patients who have had previous urinary infections and antibiotic treatment. The danger of subsequent infection with even more resistant organisms must be weighed against the presence and severity of the patient's symptoms, and the likelihood that any predisposition to infection can be overcome. It may, for example, be worthwhile to treat a *Pseudomonas* or *Klebsiella* infection which persists after removal of a temporary urinary catheter, but not to treat a similar but symptomless infection in a permanently catheterized patient.

An oral preparation called carfecillin is available, which produces modest levels of carbenicillin in urine, but not in blood. This is sometimes useful for the treatment of symptomatic *Pseudomonas* infection in a compromised bladder, but as always in such cases a permanent cure cannot be expected. Urine levels can be increased by mild restriction of fluid intake.

Follow-up
It is advisable where possible to repeat the MSU examination 1 week after the end of treatment, to confirm bacteriological cure. This is essential in children and in pregnant women.

The great majority of infections in the normal urinary tract will respond to a single course of an antibiotic to which the infecting organism is sensitive. Failure to eradicate infection after two courses of treatment is therefore an indication for intravenous urography. Infections in pregnancy are not included in this category, as the urinary tract is altered in this case by hormonal effects.

Prophylaxis
For a few patients, recurrent cystitis can cause almost permanent disability, and it is occasionally desirable to attempt prophylaxis if the predisposing cause cannot be removed. Temporary prophylaxis may be indicated in early childhood and in pregnancy to avoid ascending infection and renal damage.

A urinary antimicrobial such as nitrofurantoin may be used in a small dose or, failing this, co-trimoxazole or trimethoprim is often effective. In pregnancy, ampicillin or amoxycillin are the safest choices.

Acute pyelonephritis

Epidemiology
This is an infection of the kidney, affecting the renal pelvis, tubules and parenchyma. It is common in the altered urinary tract of pregnancy, renal cyst, ureteric stone, stricture, or congenital duplex or horseshoe kidney, but in an equal number of cases no renal abnormality is demonstrable.

The causative organisms are usually the same bacterial pathogens which affect the bladder, and infection is therefore considered to originate from ascending organisms in most cases.

Clinical features
High fever, malaise and loin pain are the rule. Distressing symptoms such as nausea, headache and shivering attacks are also common. The patient usually feels very ill. Although features of cystitis and urethritis often accompany those of pyelonephritis, this is by no means always the case, and an absence of frequency should not deter the investigator from MSU examination.

Diagnosis
MSU examination reveals the presence of many pus cells and organisms, and is almost always diagnostic. In a minority of patients the organisms can also be isolated from blood cultures, especially if these are taken during rigors.

The peripheral blood film usually shows a neutrophil leukocytosis.

Treatment
The infection may usually be treated with the same groups of antibiotics as used in cystitis, but as the parenchyma of the kidney is affected, treat-

ment of pyelonephritis should be by the parenteral route. This is even more important when blood cultures are positive. In severe infections the wide-spectrum aminoglycosides, cephalosporins or penicillins may be used, as for Gram-negative septicaemia.

Follow-up
MSU examination is advisable 1 or 2 weeks after completion of treatment. If infection persists or recurs, IVU is indicated because of the likelihood of abnormality of the renal tract. Many urologists feel that a single attack of pyelonephritis in a man or a child is an indication for IVU.

Chronic pyelonephritis

Epidemiology
In chronic pyelonephritis, as in chronic bronchitis, damage to the affected organ is followed by unavoidable recurrences of infection and further progressive tissue destruction.

The original tissue damage probably occurs during infection in the first years of life. Subsequent episodes of infection result in abscesses which block tubules, or groups of tubules, and destroy them. The kidney becomes contracted and indented by scar tissue, the tips of the medullary pyramids are lost and progressive renal failure and hypertension follow. Each infective episode is associated with severe deterioration of renal function which recovers a little less on each occasion.

Clinical features
Typically, the patient requires treatment for hypertension and may have hypertensive vascular disease and retinopathy. Episodes of symptomatic and asymptomatic infection can be detected. Fever or, in children, enuresis may be the only sign of infection, or the associated uraemia may cause drowsiness and vomiting. Anaemia and failure to thrive are common.

Diagnosis
The presence of pus cells and particularly of white cell casts in the urine is strongly suggestive. Bacteria are found during infective episodes.

The IVU may show small irregular kidneys with thinned areas of cortex and 'clubbing' of calyces where medulla has been destroyed.

Caution: analgesic nephropathy.   This is a condition which follows prolonged intake of analgesics, particularly phenacetin, but possibly also aspirin or paracetamol. White cells and casts, even fragments of renal papillae are passed in the urine, and IVU shows clubbing of calyces. A history of heavy analgesic consumption should be sought.

Treatment

The patient requires vigorous treatment of infective episodes with plentiful fluids and short courses of appropriate antibiotics. Expert management of hypertension and renal failure are required and are justified, as marked improvement usually follows control of infection.

Maintenance of high urine output is helpful in minimizing 'ascending' infections.

Acute prostatitis

This is an infection of doubtful origin which usually occurs in men below age 40. Fever, frequency, urgency and dysuria are associated with perineal, scrotal and back pain. Mucous threads are seen in terminal urine and the MSU contains pus cells and bacteria. In elderly men urinary bacteria are commonly found; in young men, chlamydiae may be responsible. Staphylococci are commonly seen.

Diagnosis is made by culture of MSU, or of prostatic secretions obtained by massage. A course of 7–10 days parenteral antibiotic is usually curative. Rarely, an abscess requires aspiration or drainage.

Acute epididymo-orchitis

Severe pain, redness and swelling of one or both sides of the scrotum are accompanied by backache, fever and neutrophil leukocytosis.

Viral infection may be responsible. Mumps is the most common and is usually characterized by parotitis and a raised serum amylase. Coxsackie infection may also cause orchitis.

Most bacterial infections are due to urinary pathogens and are associated with urinary infections or trauma to the vas deferens and epididymis. Urine culture will usually characterize the pathogen.

Brucellosis or tuberculosis can cause persistent subacute epididymo-orchitis.

Caution. Torsion of the testicle is common in boys and young men, and mimics epididymo-orchitis. If the diagnosis is in doubt immediate surgical aid should be sought.

Patients with urinary catheters

Urinary catheters can introduce infection into the urinary tract, and can precipitate bloodstream invasion by existing pathogens. They should only be used if strictly necessary and for as short a time as possible.

It is widely recognized that an indwelling catheter should empty into a sealed container, and not be left open as the lumen would quickly be invaded by bacteria. The patient should be encouraged to wash or bathe daily and to keep the perineum as clean as possible.

If a catheter must remain *in situ* for more than a week, a silicone-containing compound will cause less mucosal damage, and therefore less infection, than a plain latex one.

Regular irrigation of indwelling catheters with physiological saline (or with mild disinfectants such as noxythiolin or nitrofurazone) will remove debris which may give rise to infection or stone formation.

Drugs mentioned in this chapter

Drug	Indication	Dosage and precautions
Sulphamethizole	Domiciliary lower urinary infections; few patients,	Adult dose 200 mg five times daily, orally; child's dose a quarter to half of adult dose
Sulphafurazole	however, will adhere to such frequent dosage	Adult dose 2 g followed by 1.0 g 4–6-hourly. Child's dose is a quarter to half of the adult dose
Ampicillin ⎱ Amoxycillin ⎰	Most lower urinary tract infections	Adult dose 250–500 mg 6-hourly, orally; child's dose is a quarter to half of the adult dose. Adult dose 250 mg 8-hourly or two doses of 3.0 g 12 hours apart, orally; child's dose is a quarter to half of adult dose
Ampicillin or amoxycillin	Pyelonephritis	Adult dose 500 mg to 1.0 g 6-hourly by intramuscular or intravenous injection; child's dose 50–100 mg/kg daily in divided doses
Carfecillin	Mild bladder infection due to *Pseudomonas*	Adult dose 500 mg to 1.0 g 8-hourly, orally
Co-trimoxazole	Most lower urinary tract infections	A mixture of fixed proportions: 5 parts sulphamethoxazole to 1 part of trimethoprim; adult dose 960 mg 12-hourly, orally; child's dose is a quarter to half of adult dose
Nalidixic acid	Lower urinary tract infections Prophylaxis	Adult dose 1.0 g 6-hourly, orally for 7 days. 500 mg 6 or 12-hourly, orally; can cause nausea, diarrhoea and rashes, not recommended for children

Nitrofurantoin	Lower urinary tract infections	Adult dose 100 mg 6-hourly; nausea can be avoided by taking tablets with food
	Prophylaxis	100 mg once or twice daily; prolonged dosage can cause allergic alveolitis
Trimethoprim	Lower urinary tract infections	Adult dose 200 mg 12-hourly orally; child's dose is a quarter to half of adult dose
Other drugs	Severe pyelonephritis	Aminoglycosides, wide-spectrum penicillins or cephalosporins; see chapter 10: septicaemias and bacteraemias

9

Meningitis and Other Central Nervous System Disorders

Introduction

Several terms are used to describe various nervous system disorders attributable to infection. *Meningitis* is inflammation of the meninges surrounding the brain and spinal cord. *Encephalitis* is inflammation of the brain itself. These two conditions sometimes coexist, producing meningoencephalitis. Inflammation of the spinal cord is known as myelitis, and it can occur in encephalitis, producing encephalomyelitis.

Finally, disorders of peripheral nerves are usually called polyneuritis or polyneuropathy.

Many different pathogens can cause various combinations of these conditions (Table 6), and the patient's prognosis usually depends on the nature of the organism. It is important, therefore, to determine as early as possible the likely aetiology of the disorder because in some cases prompt treatment is essential, to save life.

Symptoms and signs of meningitis

Meningism (Fig. 16).   This is characterized by headache, neck and back stiffness and nausea. Photophobia is sometimes present, but this can also occur in other conditions associated with headache or eye disorder.

The headache is usually generalized and is the worst that the patient can remember. It is rarely abrupt in onset, though it can worsen rapidly over a few hours.

The neck and back stiffness is not always noticed by the patient, but can be demonstrated by various simple tests, including knee-kissing and Kernig's test.

Nausea is often accompanied by vomiting, especially in children.

Caution.   Children under age 2 may not show signs of neck and back stiffness even in severe meningitis. Persistent fever and vomiting are the most important signs in this age-group. Similarly, the very old may present with fever and confusion, but without meningism.

Differential diagnosis of meningism.   Meningism begins explosively in subarachnoid haemorrhage and more insidiously in malignant (e.g.

Table 6. Pathogens associated with meningitis and encephalitis

Type of pathogen	Meningitis	Encephalitis
Common viral pathogens	Mumps virus, ECHO virus, coxsackie	Mumps virus Varicella zoster (after chicken-pox)
Unusual viral pathogens	Varicella zoster, herpesvirus hominis type 2	Herpesvirus hominis type 1 Influenza virus Arboviruses Rabies virus Measles virus Rubella virus
Common bacterial pathogens	*Haemophilus influenzae* *Neisseria meningitidis* *S. pneumoniae*	
Unusual bacterial pathogens	*Listeria monocytogenes* *Streptococcus pyogenes* *Staphylococcus aureus* *Acinetobacter* species *Leptospira* species *Mycoplasma pneumoniae* *Mycobacterium tuberculosis*	*Listeria monocytogenes* *Mycoplasma pneumoniae* *Treponema pallidum* (late syphilis) *Legionella* species
Neonatal meningitis	Group B streptococcus *Escherichia coli* Other Gram-negative rods *Listeria monocytogenes*	
Rarities	*Cryptococcus neoformans* *Naegleria* ⎫ amoeba *Hartmanella* ⎬ species	*Plasmodium falciparum* *Trichinella spiralis* *Taenia* species (cysticercosis)

leukaemic) infiltration of the meninges. Mild meningism occurs without meningeal disease in acute infections such as upper lobe pneumonia, severe pharyngitis and urinary tract infections, particularly in children. In these circumstances examination of cerebrospinal fluid (CSF) is often required to elucidate the diagnosis.

Signs of raised intracranial pressure. These are unusual in most cases. Occasionally a patient with bacterial meningitis will have papilloedema. The likelihood of 'coning' after lumbar puncture must then be weighed against the need for immediate bacteriological diagnosis.

In infants, who have a patent anterior fontanelle, tension or bulging of the fontanelle appears early, and is a useful sign of meningitis.

Altered consciousness and convulsions. These signs occur only in the

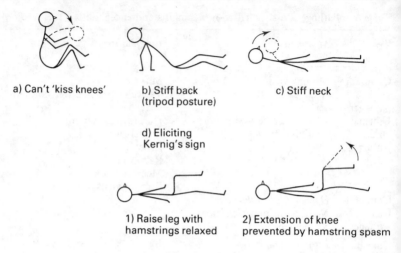

a) Can't 'kiss knees'

b) Stiff back (tripod posture)

c) Stiff neck

d) Eliciting Kernig's sign

1) Raise leg with hamstrings relaxed

2) Extension of knee prevented by hamstring spasm

Fig. 16.   Features of meningism: Kernig's test.

more severe, usually bacterial (or purulent), types of meningitis. They indicate inflammation of the underlying brain.

Symptoms and signs of encephalitis

These are the features of cerebral irritation and dysfunction. They may be associated with fever or meningism, but can exist in severe form without evidence of either.

Irritability.   Initially this takes the form of snappishness, aggressiveness and argument which may be mistaken simply for ill-nature. Physical examination at this stage will reveal exaggerated and very brisk tendon reflexes. Eventually convulsions may occur either in response to stimulation or, later, spontaneously.

Altered consciousness.   Irritability and aggressiveness are gradually replaced by drowsiness and eventually coma. Not all patients become comatose, but in those who do care must be taken to detect frequent convulsions, as the unconsciousness due to status epilepticus may be alleviated by anticonvulsant therapy.

Focal neurological signs.   The most common of these are sluggish pupillary reflexes or an extensor plantar response on one or both sides. Occasionally ptosis, squint, nystagmus or other cranial nerve deficit can occur. Many patients have no focal neurological signs.

Differential diagnosis.   Drowsiness and convulsions can occur in metabolic disorders such as uraemia, hypoglycaemia and hypocalcaemia. Various drug intoxications including those due to tricyclic antidepressants, appetite suppressants and glue solvents can also produce this state.

Laboratory investigation

Blood examination. The white blood cell count is usually low or normal in viral meningitis and encephalitis. A neutrophil leukocytosis is seen in bacterial meningitis and occasionally in mumps, especially if orchitis or pancreatitis are also present. A very high white cell count is common in pneumococcal or *Haemophilus influenzae* meningitis.

The blood glucose may be raised 1 or 2 mmol above normal in acute meningitis, and so should always be checked for comparison with the cerebrospinal fluid glucose level.

An ESR of above 75 mm in 1 hour suggests the possibility of a *Mycoplasma* infection.

Bacterial and viral cultures. Bacterial culture of CSF can provide early diagnosis, but is negative in a quarter to half of cases with purulent CSF. Blood cultures are positive in a slightly higher proportion of cases and are good evidence of the bacteriological diagnosis.

Viral culture of the CSF is less often positive, depending on the type of virus expected. A throat swab may produce a positive culture, but stools often contain virus for a longer period, and although not of direct diagnostic relation to the CSF they reflect the current viral agents existing in the patient.

Serological tests. In bacterial meningitis, counter-immunoelectrophoresis (CIE) can reveal bacterial antigens in the CSF or serum when culture has been made impossible by previous antibiotic treatment. It is of use in meningococcal, pneumococcal and *H. influenzae* meningitis.

Serological testing of the CSF (Table 7) is rarely carried out in viral infections as examination of paired blood serum samples is more reliable. For many viral and for *Mycoplasma* infections serum examination is the usual means of diagnosis.

Biopsy. Brain biopsy is the only reliable means of making a prompt diagnosis of herpes simplex encephalitis. It is not carried out in every case but, as effective antiviral drugs are developed, it is likely to be an important investigation.

Aspiration or biopsy of abscesses is sometimes carried out, and any pus obtained should be cultured.

Electroencephalography. This is seldom helpful as it tends to show generalized abnormality in both encephalitis and severe meningitis. In some cases it reveals focal abnormalities, such as bitemporal slow wave

Table 7. Summary of cerebrospinal fluid findings in nervous system disorders

	Normal	Bacterial meningitis	Viral meningitis	Encephalitis	Polyneuritis
Appearance	Clear	Opalescent or purulent	Clear	Usually clear	Clear
Cells × 10⁶/l	< 6 All lymphocytes	Often > 500 Neutrophils ? bacteria	Often 20–100 Neutros early; usually lymphos	Normal or excess lymphos	Normal
Protein (g/l)	0.1–0.4	Often > 0.9	0.5–0.9 usually	Normal or up to 1.0	Normal early, can rise greatly later
Glucose (mmol/l)	0.5–1.5 below blood level	Reduced, can be 0.0	Normal (may be low in mumps)	Normal	Normal

patterns, which are seen in herpes simplex encephalitis but are not diagnostic.

Scanning techniques. Isotope or computerized scanning may reveal intracranial abscesses. The computerized scan can also demonstrate hydrocephalus at an early stage. Areas of oedema can be seen in encephalitis; in herpes simplex encephalitis the temporal lobes are often abnormal. Tuberculomas have a typical appearance on computerized scanning.

General management of patients with CNS disease
While a great many patients with mild disease require only minimum nursing care a few, who are restless and disorientated, present a severe nursing problem. A few points are worth remembering:

1. acute retention of urine is common and adds greatly to distress and restlessness;
2. frequent epileptic seizures can exacerbate drowsiness and confusion;
3. sedative drugs are relatively ineffective in severely excitable patients.

The best course of action is often to enclose the patient in a comfortable bed with secure cot sides, to avoid restraint, to rearrange the patient and associated catheters and infusion lines only when unavoidable, and to give minimal sedation. If restlessness or convulsions are exhausting the patient a chlormethiazole infusion, titrated to produce light sleep, can be extremely helpful. Diazepam carries the risk of producing severe respiratory depression or paradoxical aggression, and repeated doses can be cumulative. Chlorpromazine is a good sedative but, on rare occasions, exacerbates epilepsy.

Viral meningitis

Epidemiology
Viral meningitis is a common illness which is often associated with infection by respiratory agents or with enterovirus infections. It is usually transmitted by droplets or by the faecal–oral route. The incidence of meningitis is related to the epidemic incidence of these viruses, particularly to ECHOvirus epidemics.

Clinical features
The typical features of a viral infection are associated with the occurrence of meningism, which usually follows the appearance of other symptoms. In a few cases however, and mumps is an example, meningitis may precede or coexist with the other features. A macular rash in enterovirus

infection or the parotitis of mumps sometimes give strong indication of the diagnosis.

Patients with viral meningitis are rarely disorientated even if the fever and meningism are severe. There is, however, an overlap between meningitis and encephalitis, and excessive drowsiness should prompt a search for evidence of encephalitis.

Diagnosis
Lumbar puncture is the diagnostic procedure and should be carried out in all but the mildest cases, to confirm the viral aetiology. One important diagnosis which can be confused with that of viral meningitis is tuberculous meningitis, which presents a similar CSF picture in its earliest stages (see below).

Cultures of CSF, throat swabs and stool may reveal the responsible pathogen. Examination of paired sera will sometimes provide a retrospective diagnosis by showing a significant rise in antibody levels. Pathologists usually test routinely for a variety of common viral pathogens if requested to investigate a case of viral meningitis.

Treatment
Bedrest and adequate analgesic medication are usually all that is required. Antiemetic drugs are effective in alleviating vomiting.

Most patients recover from their fever and meningism within a few days to a week. If they deteriorate or fail to improve during this time the diagnosis should be reconsidered and lumbar puncture may be repeated.

Fatigue and headaches may persist for some weeks after the fever and meningism have subsided.

Poliomyelitis

Epidemiology
This is a disease in which viral meningitis is associated with inflammation and destruction of lower motor neurones in the brainstem and spinal cord. It is usually due to infection with one of the three serotypes of poliovirus and spreads mainly by the faecal–oral route, particularly via sewage-contaminated water. Some rare cases are associated with coxsackie or other enterovirus infections.

In developed countries immunization against poliomyelitis is now readily available but elderly people, and children whose parents refuse or neglect immunization can contract the disease. Large endemic areas still exist in some countries, and travellers to these areas may be exposed to infection. In the endemic areas, natural immunity is acquired early, so that poliomyelitis is predominantly a disease of young children.

Clinical features
The incubation period is 10–14 days (range 3–35 days). A typical

enterovirus pharyngitis and sometimes mild diarrhoea then occurs. In a proportion of patients viral meningitis develops and a minority of these cases have myelitis with sufficient lower motor neurone damage to develop clinical paralysis.

Paralysis is flaccid and asymmetrical. There is never any sensory deficit and hardly ever an abnormal plantar reflex. The shoulder girdle, anterior tibial and trunk muscles are most often affected. Bulbar paralysis may lead to disorders of speech, swallowing and breathing. Recovery of power begins after a delay of 2 or 3 weeks and may be complete, especially in children. Bulbar palsy often recovers well. Improvement in strength can continue for up to 2 years.

The development of paralysis is more likely in men and in pregnant women. It can also occur after vigorous exercise, after recent trauma including minor operations, and in muscles recently affected by intramuscular injections.

Diagnosis
Lumbar puncture reveals typical changes of viral meningitis in the CSF during the 'meningitis' and the 'early paralytic' stages. Virus may be isolated from stools and less often from CSF or throat swabs. Virus excretion in the stools can persist for 6–12 weeks after the acute illness.

Neutralizing or precipitating antibodies can be detected in rising titres in paired sera.

Treatment
For non-paralytic cases this is the same as for any viral meningitis. For paralytic cases, bedrest and avoidance of fatigue or trauma are continued for 5–7 days after the temperature has fallen to normal. When bulbar or respiratory paralysis occur, tube feeding or assisted ventilation may be required. Measurement of the vital capacity gives a good indication of respiratory muscle function.

The remainder of the treatment consists of graded physiotherapy to assist return of function. Bulbar and respiratory paralysis almost always improve, but other weakness may persist, especially in adults.

Prophylaxis
Both a live attenuated (Sabin) and a killed (Salk) vaccine are available, and can be given in childhood. It may be worthwhile giving the live vaccine (OPV, oral polio vaccine) to those at risk in an epidemic, for the vaccine strain might compete with the virulent virus and prevent some infections.

Meningococcal meningitis

Epidemiology
Neisseria meningitidis, a Gram-negative coccus, is a resident of the

pharynx and a fluctuating number of carriers is present in any population. Some people who acquire meningococci in the pharynx go on to develop meningitis. Those most susceptible are children aged 18 months to 5 years and adolescents aged 15–25 years, who have low or absent antibody levels. Outbreaks sometimes occur in large groups of susceptible individuals, such as military recruits. About one-tenth of all cases have a history of contact with a previous case.

Meningococci can be placed into three main serogroups; A, B and C, and less commonly X, Y, Z and W135. Group B is the major epidemic strain in Europe at present, but in tropical countries other groups may be prevalent. Sporadic illness may be caused by any group.

Clinical features

The incubation period is variable, but is thought to be only a few days. Some secondary cases have occurred up to 3 weeks after contact. Severe illness can develop in a matter of hours with high fever, severe meningism and rapid development of confusion, coma, shock and death in a few hours. In the majority of cases the clinical picture develops within 24–36 hours.

Nine-tenths of patients have a petechial rash, which is occasionally preceded by a transient macular eruption. The petechiae may be small and sparse, even confined to the conjunctivae, but the extensor surfaces are susceptible to more severe ecchymotic lesions, which may have necrotic centres. The rash is associated with slight reduction of the platelet count and fibrinogen levels, indicating mild disseminated intravascular coagulation (DIC).

Unusual accompaniments of meningococcal disease include endocarditis, myocarditis, ophthalmitis, septic arthritis of large joints and, in fulminating cases, bilateral adrenal haemorrhage (Waterhouse–Friderichsen syndrome).

Diagnosis

Lumbar puncture reveals typical CSF changes of bacterial meningitis. Gram-negative diplococci may be seen both free and within the white cells. Culture of the CSF allows confirmation of the diagnosis. Blood cultures are also likely to be positive.

Meningococcal antigen may be detectable by CIE of serum or CSF even after antibiotic therapy.

Treatment

This should be commenced *without delay*. The treatment of choice is intravenous benzylpenicillin, which quickly passes the damaged blood brain barrier. In meningococcal disease no added advantage is gained by giving intrathecal antibiotics. Although cure has been recorded after a single intravenous injection, many specialists prefer to give large doses for 3–5 days. Chloramphenicol is the drug of second choice, while cephalosporins have proved rather disappointing though cefuroxime may be an exception to this. Sulphonamides are not usually used because 20–25% of commonly seen meningococci are sulphonamide-resistant.

The alterations in platelet and fibrinogen levels respond promptly to the antibiotic treatment, and there is no evidence of any advantage in heparin therapy. In rare cases platelet transfusion or administration of blood products may be required.

Mortality, even with treatment, is 9–15%.

Complications
Sudden neurological catastrophe.   This can occur either during illness or when the patient is apparently improving. Often due to a vascular lesion in the brainstem it causes respiratory or cardiorespiratory dysfunction or arrest. The outlook for resuscitation and recovery is bleak.

Reactive effusions.   These occur late, after 7–10 days, often affecting the knees. A serous effusion contains many leukocytes but no bacteria. Spontaneous recovery occurs over several days, and only symptomatic treatment is required. Pericardial or pleural effusion is less common.

General complications of meningitis.   These include irritability, cranial nerve deficits commonly affecting the second, fourth, sixth or eighth nerves, and hydrocephalus with raised intracranial pressure.

Prophylaxis
Immunization is available against group A and C meningococci, but not against group B.

When a case occurs, it is reasonable to offer antibiotic prophylaxis to domestic or dormitory contacts who have prolonged daily exposure to the patient. The intention is to eradicate the virulent meningococcus from the contacts and treatment should not be delayed to await throat swabs, or typing of the organism as the natural presence of carriers in any population will confuse such investigations. Penicillin will not affect the carrier state. The drug of choice for prophylaxis is sulphadiazine (other sulphonamides are less effective). If the meningococcus is sulphonamide-resistant or its sensitivities are unknown, rifampicin can be used. Minocycline is also of use, though it has unpleasant side-effects (Table 8).

Pneumococcal meningitis

Epidemiology
This illness tends to affect adults. The pneumococcus is a resident of the pharynx and is also found in the paranasal sinuses and in the infected middle ear. Predispositions to the development of meningitis include chronic sinusitis, nasal polypectomy, chronic otitis media, recent head

Table 8.   Chemoprophylaxis of meningococcal disease

When the organism causing the original case is suphonamide-sensitive	Sulphadiazine Adult dose 1.0 g twice daily orally for two days; age 1–12 years 500 mg twice daily; age 3–12 months 250 mg twice daily
When the organism causing the original case is sulphonamide-resistant	Rifampicin Adult dose 600 mg twice daily orally for 2 days (not recommended in pregnancy); age 1–12 years 10 mg/kg twice daily; age 3–12 months 5 mg/kg twice daily (Minocycline may be used if rifampicin cannot be but like other tetracyclines it is deposited in growing teeth and bones. It also causes nausea, dizziness and vertigo. Adult dose 200 mg orally, then 100 mg 12 hourly)

NOTE   In Canada and the United States rifampicin prophylaxis is used for contacts of *H. influenzae* meningitis cases. In the United Kingdom the incidence of such infections is lower and the balance between the risk of infection and of severe side-effects of the medication is less clear.

injury, chronic CSF rhinorrhoea, and alcoholism. Patients with predispositions, especially CSF leaks, may have recurrent attacks of meningitis.

Clinical features
The features of meningitis develop over 24–48 hours, often following exacerbation of a predisposing factor. The ears, nose and cranium should be examined for evidence of suppuration or CSF leak. Testing with glucose-measuring strips will give a positive result if a nasal discharge contains CSF.

Diagnosis
CSF microscopy and culture, blood culture and CIE for pneumococcal antigen in CSF and serum can contribute to the diagnosis.

Treatment
The treatment of choice is high-dose intravenous benzylpenicillin which should be continued for 7–10 days. Chloramphenicol is an effective alternative, and the narrow-spectrum cephalosporins have been found useful.

If the patient fails to make progress it is worth using a scanning technique to exclude the possibility of intracranial or intracerebral abscess, which may require drainage.

When the meningitis has been treated, surgical management of skull defects, or intracranial suppuration, may be necessary.

Complications

Abscess formation, cranial nerve defects and intellectual impairment are more common than with other organisms. The incidence of recurrent meningitis is significant. Mortality is high, averaging 20% and is closely related to the age of the patient.

Haemophilus influenzae meningitis

Haemophilus influenzae is a Gram-negative rod which is a resident of the upper respiratory tract. It causes meningitis in infants, mostly between age 3 months and 3 years. Meningism develops insidiously over several days following the appearance of upper respiratory symptoms.

It is often difficult to discern the organism on CSF smears, but CSF and blood cultures, or CIE of CSF and serum may reveal the diagnosis.

The treatment of choice is chloramphenicol given for 10–14 days. Increasing numbers of *H.influenzae* isolates are resistant to ampicillin. Cefuroxime has been given in high doses and has been a satisfactory treatment in some cases.

Purulent meningitis of obscure aetiology

As many as a quarter of cases of severe meningitis with neutrophil leukocytosis in the blood, neutrophil pleiocytosis in the CSF and low CSF glucose, are resistant to diagnosis by microscopy, culture or by serological techniques.

Although no bacterial pathogen is detectable, the disease is almost certainly bacterial meningitis. The treatment most appropriate to common bacterial pathogens is chloramphenicol, which is effective against them all. Although some physicians like to add two or three other antibiotics, the combination of chloramphenicol, a bacteriostatic agent, with bacteriocidal antibiotics has theoretical disadvantages.

High-dose cefuroxime may offer an alternative to chloramphenicol in this difficult situation, but experience in its use is limited.

Unusual types of meningitis

Meningitis in patients with CSF shunts. An increasing number of patients with CSF shunts and valves is seen, as treatment of hydrocephalus becomes more widely available. The usual shunts are ventriculocaval and ventriculoperitoneal. Patients with shunts occasionally suffer a 'spontaneous' attack of meningitis and in a large proportion of these cases *Staph.epidermidis* is recovered from the CSF or the shunt itself. Blood cultures may be negative.

The majority of *Staph.epidermidis* isolates are resistant to benzylpenicillin, and must be treated with high doses of cloxacillin or flucloxacillin, which may be combined with fusidic acid as in staphylococcal septicaemia.

Acinetobacter spp. (formerly *Mima polymorpha*).   This Gram-negative organism, with variable morphology, is capable of causing septicaemia and endocarditis. It is an unusual cause of purulent meningitis but it is important to bear in mind, as it can mimic meningococcal meningitis and produce a petechial rash. The similarity may extend to the appearances on Gram-stained CSF.

It is not usually sensitive to benzylpenicillin or even to chloramphenicol. Aminoglycosides, or very wide-spectrum penicillins and cephalosporins are likely to be required for effective treatment.

Streptococcus pyogenes and *Staphylococcus aureus.*   These organisms sometimes cause meningitis as part of a Gram-positive septicaemia. Blood and CSF cultures are almost always positive, and antibiotic treatment may be chosen on the basis of sensitivity testing. The appropriate penicillin is the drug of first choice.

Listeria monocytogenes.   This is a Gram-positive rod, widespread in the environment and in animals. It can be confused with diphtheroids and *Erysipelothrix*. It tends to affect neonates, or those over middle age with debilitating disease. It is sensitive to ampicillin, erythromycin and chloramphenicol.

Leptospira spp.   Meningitis due to these organisms may occur alone or combined with more widespread manifestations (see Chapter 7). The presence of conjunctivitis or abnormal liver function is a helpful clue in some cases. Leptospirosis is notoriously resistant to antibiotic therapy, but large doses of benzylpenicillin may be helpful.

Cryptococcal meningitis.   This is a rare but recognized condition which complicates some disorders of cell-mediated immunity. It occurs in patients with Hodgkin's disease, other lymphomas, and some types of leukaemia.

An illness with fever and meningism develops over several days, sometimes more acutely, and the patient appears clinically to have bacterial meningitis. Lumbar puncture reveals the yeast-like cells of *Cryptococcus neoformans* in the CSF of about half of cases. Culture of the organism and detection of cryptococcal antigen in the CSF is more likely to reveal the diagnosis.

Treatment is with amphotericin given by daily intravenous infusion and there is a good chance of response if an early diagnosis is made, though relapses or second attacks can occur. Flucytosine may be combined with amphotericin, but should not be used alone, as the yeasts will quickly become resistant to it.

Amoebic meningitis. This is an extremely rare condition due to invasion of the meninges by free-living amoebae of the *Naegleria* or *Hartmanella* species. These amoebae are found in warm, muddy water (puddles, hot springs or unchlorinated swimming facilities) and appear to enter the meninges via the cribriform plate during swimming or water accidents.

The meningitis is similar to severe bacterial meningitis, but amoebae can be seen among the polymorphs on fresh CSF smears. No effective treatment is known and the outcome is usually fatal.

Fungal meningitis. This is usually a complication of fungal septicaemia in a patient with severe immune deficiency. Most often due to *Candida spp.* it is associated with large or multiple abscesses and occlusion of blood vessels by septic thrombi. Treatment is with amphotericin, but the outlook is very poor.

Neonatal meningitis

This is often an intrapartum infection derived from contact with organisms in the mother's urine or faeces. Group B streptococci, *E. coli*, other Enterobacteriaceae and occasionally salmonellae are the types of organism involved. Diagnosis is made by lumbar puncture or ventricular puncture. High-dose penicillin is used to treat group B streptococcal disease. Treatment with aminoglycosides or the latest wide-spectrum penicillins or cephalosporins may need to be given for two weeks or more in Gram-negative infections. The intrathecal as well as the intravenous route may be used in these cases, to ensure high antibiotic levels in the CSF.

Mortality is high and neurological sequelae are common.

Cerebral abscesses

Abscesses can occur after meningitis, after head injury, as extensions of sepsis in the ears or sinuses, or apparently spontaneously (but presumably after bacteraemia). They can appear in the brain substance or in blocked-off ventricles.

Bacteriological investigation almost always reveals a mixture of micro-aerophilic streptococci, for example *Streptococcus milleri*, and *Bacteroides spp.* The CSF often shows a high protein level and a pleiocytosis with many lymphocytes and a few neutrophils.

The best treatment is surgical drainage or enucleation of the abscess under antibiotic cover. Inaccessible abscesses or ventricular abscesses are sometimes amenable to high-dose antibiotic therapy with benzyl-penicillin or cefuroxime plus metronidazole. Intravenous medication is usually continued for at least 3 or 4 weeks but even then ventricular abscesses (ventriculitis) have a high mortality.

Tuberculous meningitis

Epidemiology
Tuberculous meningitis is often a manifestation of primary tuberculosis, especially following a primary contact in children and adolescents. Occasionally it accompanies severe cavitating or disseminated infection. The tubercle bacilli probably reach the meninges via the bloodstream.

Clinical features
These are very variable. Sometimes the onset is insidious with variable headache, personality change or minor neurological deficit. In other cases the course is similar to that of acute meningitis.

In untreated cases cranial nerve lesions, hydrocephalus and paraplegia can develop quite suddenly, so that early suspicion and diagnosis are important if grave complications are to be avoided.

Diagnosis
This can be very difficult. Lumbar puncture offers the best opportunity. Although the CSF appears clear and often contains only a minor excess of lymphocytes, the glucose level is usually low and the protein level rather high. A thorough search for alcohol-acid fast bacteria is best carried out by an expert.

A second lumbar puncture may be necessary, and will show a further fall in glucose and rapid rise in protein levels.

The tuberculin test is not always positive initially, but becomes so quite suddenly and is worth repeating after 7–10 days.

The chest X-ray may show a typical tuberculous lesion.

Treatment
This should be commenced on reasonable suspicion and should not be delayed pending cultural confirmation of diagnosis. Standard triple therapy with rifampicin, isoniazid and ethambutol (see Chapter 13) is satisfactory, but many physicians like to add pyrazinamide, which readily penetrates the blood–brain barrier, at least for the first 2–3 months. Doses of the standard drugs can be doubled for the first 2 or 3 weeks. Treatment is usually continued with rifampicin and isoniazid (plus pyridoxine supplements) for 12–18 months, depending on response.

If early focal neurological deficit occurs, prednisolone added to the regimen may reduce inflammation and minimize permanent damage. Quite gross paraparesis and other lesions sometimes resolve very well with combined prednisolone and multiple therapy, but there is little hope of resolution if treatment is delayed.

Intrathecal medication is rarely indicated, though hydrocortisone can be given by this route if the need is acute.

Myelography is indicated if spinal symptoms occur, as decompression of tuberculous obstructing lesions is often possible.

Computerized brain scanning will detect progressive hydrocephalus, and reveal the need for shunting or drainage of CSF.

Caution. Tuberculous meningitis can be difficult to distinguish from partially treated bacterial meningitis, in which lymphocytes replace polymorphs in the CSF. It is occasionally necessary to treat a patient for both conditions while diagnostic procedures are carried out.

Encephalitis

Epidemiology
Many viral infections can be accompanied by mild or trivial encephalitis (infective encephalitis) or followed by it (postinfectious encephalitis). The majority of cases, even if severe, are self-limiting within 1 or 2 weeks. In Europe herpes simplex is the most common severe encephalitis, usually caused by Herpesvirus hominis type 1. In the Americas, Japan, Russia and Australia arbovirus encephalitis also occurs. The arboviruses exist in wild birds or small mammals and are transmitted to man (and horses) by mosquitoes during the warmer months of the year.

Clinical features
These are the features of increasing cerebral irritation and dysfunction. In herpes simplex encephalitis fever is trivial or even absent, while in arbovirus infections it is usually marked and may be accompanied by meningism.

The finding of mucocutaneous herpes simplex in a patient with encephalitis may be a useful pointer to the diagnosis, but occurs in rather less than half of cases (and is common also after pneumococcal and meningococcal infections).

Signs of raised intracranial pressure are not the rule, but occur in a few severe cases who develop cerebral oedema. Engorgement of the retinal veins is not uncommon, but does not always presage papilloedema.

As with meningitis, signs of encephalitis are few in infants. Listlessness, screaming, bulging fontanelle and perhaps convulsions are the most helpful clues.

Diagnosis
The white blood cell count is not characteristically altered. The pleiocytosis and protein elevation in the CSF is very variable, and usually much less marked in herpes simplex than in arbovirus encephalitis.

Examination of brain biopsy material can permit an early diagnosis of herpes simplex encephalitis but serological techniques performed on CSF are unreliable. The majority of cases have bitemporal abnormalities in the EEG, but these may also be seen in other encephalitides. A rising titre of antibodies to herpes simplex in paired sera will confirm the diagnosis.

Most arbovirus encephalitides can be diagnosed by the demonstration of specific antibodies in the serum early in the illness. Haemagglutination-inhibiting (HAI) antibodies are convenient and frequently used.

Treatment
This is symptomatic and supportive as described in the introduction. Dexamethasone is useful in alleviating raised intracranial pressure, but has no effect on the encephalitis itself.

There is a chance that early treatment with antiviral agents will improve the prognosis of herpes simplex encephalitis. Vidarabine and cytarabine probably have a slight effect, but hopes for significant activity rest on the new drug acyclovir. To be useful, treatment should be commenced early in the course of disease, immediately after brain biopsy if this is carried out.

Follow-up
After herpes simplex of encephalitis sequelae are relatively common, occurring in up to half of patients in some series. Personality changes, epilepsy, paresis and cranial nerve dysfunction are the commonest long-term effects.

Rabies

This is an almost uniformly fatal encephalomyelitis which is transmitted by inoculation of saliva from an infected animal. Carnivores, especially wolves and dogs, suffer a 'furious' form of the disease and readily transmit it by biting. Other animals have 'dumb' rabies and may be listless and paralysed. Humans most often develop the excitable form.

Because the inoculated virus enters the peripheral nerves and invades the CNS by retrograde spread, the incubation period varies from 10 days to a year or more, depending on whether the bite or scratch was proximal or distal to the CNS. Eventually pain and paraesthesia at the inoculation site are followed by excitability, severe painful pharyngeal and laryngeal spasms, producing apparent fear of water (hydrophobia) and later by paralysis and death.

Effective prophylaxis is available and except in regularly exposed individuals is given after exposure:
1. the wound should be washed with soap or disinfectant,
2. a course of human diploid cell rabies vaccine should be given,
3. human antirabies globulin should be given as soon as possible after exposure, to destroy viruses in the tissues and bloodstream.

Other types of vaccine are much inferior to the diploid cell preparation and should soon be replaced by it in all countries.

If the animal concerned is well 2 weeks after the incident, it was almost certainly not infectious at the initial encounter. Many European owners have their pets immunized and possess certificates of vaccination.

Subacute sclerosing panencephalitis (SSPE)

This is a rare and fatal infection due to a measles virus. A child who had measles in the first 2 years of life, after an average 6 or 7 years' interval, becomes clumsy and inattentive. The disease progresses over a period of months or years, first via a stage of myoclonic attacks with associated EEG abnormalities and finally to spasticity, decerebration and death. No effective treatment has been discovered.

Benign myalgic encephalomyelitis (Royal Free disease)

This controversial disease entity was postulated after an epidemic in which patients had a feverish illness with elements of meningism, various neurological disturbances, CSF abnormalities and abnormal muscle function. A few progressed to have chronic neurological disability and muscle fatigue. No aetiology is recognized and the disorder is notoriously resistant to any treatment.

Ascending polyneuritis (Guillain–Barré disease)

Epidemiology
The aetiology of this disorder is unknown, but three-quarters of patients have a history of respiratory or gastrointestinal illness 1 or 2 weeks before its onset. Known associations exist between Guillain-Barré disease and atypical pneumonias, cytomegalovirus infection and vaccination. The middle-aged and elderly are most commonly affected.

Clinical features
Weakness and paraesthesiae in the legs occur in all patients, though objective sensory loss may be difficult to demonstrate. Tendon reflexes are lost. Paralysis often progresses for 1–2 weeks, sometimes longer, and ascends to involve trunk, sphincters, arms, respiratory muscles and cranial nerves in the most severe cases. About half of patients suffer sufficient reduction in vital capacity to require artificial ventilation. Facial palsy occurs in about half of patients and is closely correlated with respiratory insufficiency.

Urinary and respiratory infections are common in the severely paralysed but, even in the oldest patients, mortality is extremely low and recovery usually occurs, though it may take several weeks.

Treatment
This is entirely supportive. Corticosteroids have been given to some patients without definite evidence of benefit. Regular measurement of vital capacity gives a good indication of the progress of respiratory muscle function.

A few chronic cases have responded well to plasma exchange.

Drugs mentioned in this chapter

Drug	Indication	Usage and precautions
Acyclovir	Herpes simplex and varicella zoster infections	Dose for all ages 10 mg/kg 8-hourly by slow intravenous infusion; do not give over less than 1 hour. Check blood urea, it may rise if drug is infused too quickly or if dosage is too high
Benzylpenicillin	Pneumococcal, meningococcal and streptococcal meningitis; gentamicin may be added for group B streptococci	Adult dose 1.2–3.0 g (2–5 mega units) 4 to 6-hourly intra-venously (average = 3 or 4 mega units 4-hourly); child's dose is a quarter to half of adult dose; neonates will often tolerate up to 600 mg (1 mega unit) 4-hourly; overdosage can cause reversible hyperexcitability, confusion or convulsions
Cefuroxime	Purulent meningitis (alternative drug)	Adult dose 3.0–4.5 g 6-hourly by intravenous infusion; child's dose 200 mg/kg daily in divided doses
Chloramphenicol	*H. influenzae* meningitis and purulent meningitis of unknown cause	Adult dose 2.0–3.0 g daily in three or four doses orally or intravenously; child's dose 50–100 mg/kg daily in divided doses; *not recommended for neonates*, but 25 mg/kg daily can be given if imperative; dosage must be stopped if shock develops
Gentamicin	Neonatal Gram-negative meningitis	Neonatal dose 3 mg/kg 12-hourly by intramuscular injection; intrathecal therapy: dose is 1 mg daily with 2–4 mg/kg daily, by intramuscular injection, in three divided doses
Latamoxef	Wide-spectrum including anaerobes, resists penicillase	Adult dose 3.0–12.0 g daily in three 8-hourly doses by intra-muscular or intravenous injection; child's dose 50 mg/kg 12-hourly; infant age 1–4 weeks 25 mg/kg 8-hourly; infant up to age 1 week 25 mg/kg 12-hourly

Human diploid cell rabies vaccine and human rabies immunoglobulin	Postexposure prophylaxis of rabies	These preparations are held in stock by some Public Health Laboratories; they can be obtained by contacting any Public Health Laboratory, when arrangements will be made for their prompt despatch
Vidarabine	Herpes simplex and varicella zoster infections	Dose for all ages is 10 mg/kg daily by intravenous infusion; dose should be reduced in renal impairment and reduced or discontinued if the blood count falls

10

Septicaemias and Bacteraemias

Introduction

Septicaemia is a condition in which bacteria, or occasionally fungi, are multiplying in the bloodstream. It differs from bacteraemia, in which organisms exist transiently in the blood after entering the vascular system from a local infection or via a penetrating injury. There is, however, an indistinct division between the two conditions, which may alternate or overlap.

Blood has many formed and soluble components, including phagocytes, lymphocytes, immunoglobulins and complement, which contribute to its natural bacteriocidal properties. Bacteraemia is usually quickly terminated because of these properties but if natural defences are overwhelmed it can lead to septicaemia or to metastatic infections.

Routes of infection

Through skin defects.   Small cuts or grazes, chickenpox lesions, injection sites, traumatic lacerations and surgical incisions can all admit skin organisms to the bloodstream. Recognized examples of this are *Streptococcus pyogenes* septicaemia following a cut or graze, and *Staphylococcus aureus* septicaemia in intravenous drug abusers or complicating chickenpox. Septicaemia may also be acquired if a skin lesion is contaminated by soil or by animal teeth and claws.

From an existing infectious focus.   In a small proportion of cases of pneumonia, pyogenic abscess, cholecystitis, pyelonephritis or other infections, bacteraemia overwhelms the blood's defences and septicaemia follows. The nature of the organism in the blood may be deduced from the site of the original focus of infection.

Following surgery or trauma.   If the bowel is opened or perforated, faecal organisms will contaminate the adjacent peritoneum and wound. In a proportion of patients bloodstream invasion and Gram-negative septicaemia follows.   Instrumentation such as cystoscopy, culdoscopy, pancreatic and biliary intubation or cardiac catheterization are all known to entail some risk of bacteraemia. The risk is increased if the site to be examined is already infected. Following examination of the infected bladder or the inflamed pancreas, bacteraemia and septicaemia are recognized as significant hazards.

Effect of immunodeficiency. In immunodeficiency bacteraemia cannot easily be terminated by blood defences. Normally non-pathogenic commensal or environmental organisms can then cause septicaemias which demand vigorous antibiotic therapy. Eventuallly, because of altered body defences and repeated antibiotic therapy, multiply-resistant Gram-negative organisms displace other organisms from the skin, the gut and the dental clefts. Recurrent septicaemias due to *Pseudomonas*, *Klebsiella* and *Serratia* species are often the end result in such cases.

Features of Gram-positive septicaemias
There are few specific features to suggest a diagnosis of Gram-positive septicaemia. The illness often begins insidiously with high fever and increasing malaise. Non-specific symptoms such as headache, nausea, vomiting and diarrhoea indicate the severity of the illness rather than its origin. Sometimes a typical skin rash will help to identify the causative organism. Shock is uncommon as a presenting feature, though it can appear suddenly in the terminal stages and it then indicates a poor prognosis.

In spite of apparent cardiovascular stability, renal function is often impaired. A surprisingly high blood urea and poorly concentrated urine, even if the urine output appears satisfactory, are helpful indicators of potentially serious disease.

In rare cases, disseminated intravascular coagulation (DIC) occurs and may cause confusion with meningococcal and other Gram-negative septicaemias.

Features of Gram-negative septicaemias
Septicaemias due to Gram-negative rods are associated with the presence of endotoxin in the blood. Endotoxin is a lipopolysaccharide which forms part of the cell-wall structure of the bacilli. Its release in the bloodstream results in shock and tissue damage, the consequences of which can determine the ultimate prognosis.

Endotoxic shock. Loss of vascular tone and leakage of fluid through increasingly permeable vascular endothelium results in a profound fall in the blood pressure. The blood volume may be increased, in which case the patient often has a pink skin, or decreased causing peripheral cyanosis and skin pallor. In either case capillary circulation is sluggish and the jugular venous pressure is low.

Reduced tissue perfusion is quickly followed by falling urine output and rising blood creatinine.

Pulmonary oedema.   This is due to increased permeability of the alveolar capillary endothelium. In severe cases protein and red blood cells enter the alveoli and an appearance of hyaline membrane (adult respiratory distress syndrome or ARDS) develops.

The pulmonary oedema impairs gas exchange and combines with shock and reduced perfusion to produce severe tissue anoxia.

Lactic acidosis.   This is not a common condition, but it occurs particularly in septicaemic patients with pre-existing hepatic or renal disease, and in diabetics taking biguanide drugs. Rapid and deep breathing (Kussmaul respiration) is characteristic, but is also seen in diabetic ketoacidosis which must be excluded by estimation of urine glucose and ketones, and of blood glucose.

In lactic acidosis the blood bicarbonate level is very low, often below 5 mmol/l, and if the blood lactate is estimated, it is usually more than twice the upper limit of normal.

Disseminated intravascular coagulation (DIC).   The blood coagulation pathways may be set in progress by damage to vascular endothelium, by direct action of endotoxin or by interaction between clotting factors, immune complexes and complement. The result is the formation of fibrin within the vascular tree. Intravascular fibrin is normally broken down by plasmins, but when this mechanism is saturated, small thrombi form in the blood vessels.

Rapid formation of fibrin depletes blood fibrinogen levels, while plasmin activity produces excess fibrin degradation products (FDPs). The blood becomes incoagulable, and widespread bleeding occurs with platelet utilization and depletion.

The clinical picture is of a patient with petechiae, bruising and prolonged oozing from venepuncture sites. Fibrin thrombi occlude small blood vessels causing patchy necrotic areas which are seen on the skin. In severe cases there may be haematuria and bleeding from mucous membranes.

General management of septicaemia

Blood cultures, urine, pus, wound swabs and a serum sample are collected as quickly as possible.

The first principle of management is to commence effective resuscitation and chemotherapy without delay. If clinical findings indicate the nature of the septicaemia, then the choice of therapy may be straightforward. If there are no clinical clues, wide-spectrum agents or a mixture of agents may be required until the organism and its sensitivities have been identified.

If infection is spreading from an enclosed focus such as an abscess, or from an obstructed viscus such as the gallbladder, surgical drainage may be necessary to achieve a cure. Surgery is best carried out when the patient has therapeutic blood levels of antibiotics. This provides some protection against any bacteria entering the bloodstream during operation. Blood levels of most antibiotics can be estimated by a microbiologist, if required. Even simple measures, like relieving retention of infected urine, can be sufficient to terminate a bacteraemia and should not be neglected.

Management of shock. The first essential is to give enough fluid to fill the vascular bed. The nature of the fluid is relatively unimportant; electrolyte solutions are just as acceptable as plasma expanders in the emergency situation. For maintenance of blood pressure, plasma protein fraction (PPF) is recommended as it is not lost from the vascular bed and it may help to attract oedema fluid out of the tissues.

Inotropic agents may be used if fluid therapy alone does not restore blood pressure, or if the central venous pressure rises (above 8–10 cm of water) during fluid administration without a response in the blood pressure. Dopamine is the drug of choice as it increases cardiac output and renal perfusion, but does not cause vasoconstriction unless given in high doses. Isoprenaline is an acceptable alternative, but may cause cardiac dysrrhythmias.

Corticosteroids are often given as there is evidence that they reduce the effect of endotoxin on neutrophils and vascular endothelium. Intravenous hydrocortisone or methylprednisolone are the usual drugs of choice.

Vasodilators, particularly hydralazine and sodium nitroprusside, have been recommended by some physicians who find that they improve peripheral perfusion in patients with gross cyanosis and vasoconstriction. They seem to increase cardiac output by removing the increased peripheral resistance to blood flow ('afterload reduction').

Management of pulmonary oedema. This is extremely difficult in the face of low blood pressure and low urine output. Intravenous frusemide or bumetanide may promote renal function if the blood pressure is restored, but has little effect on the original haemodynamic problem.

It may be worthwhile giving a vasodilator drug in the hope of transferring excess fluid from the pulmonary to the newly dilated systemic vascular bed. This makes good scientific sense and often has a measure of success.

If other measures fail, positive pressure ventilation, particularly positive end-expiratory pressure (PEEP), can move fluid from the alveoli to the circulation by a hydrostatic effect. High concentrations of inspired oxygen can be given at the same time, and may relieve tissue anoxia.

Management of lactic acidosis. This very serious condition can prove intractable even when the septicaemia has been controlled. The mainstay of treatment is the neutralization of acidosis with large intravenous doses of bicarbonate. Many patients require 50–100 mmol per hour, or more, before any benefit is seen. Doses of this size impose a very large sodium and water load on the failing cardiovascular system, and can limit the usefulness of treatment.

Recent claims for the use of sodium nitroprusside infusion have been impressive. It is thought that improved tissue perfusion reverses anoxia and terminates lactate production, allowing modest doses of bicarbonate to elevate the blood pH.

Management of DIC.   This condition usually responds quite quickly to removal of the underlying cause, with restoration of platelet levels and clotting factors over a matter of 12–24 hours. Platelet infusions or plasma components can be given if severe bleeding threatens during this time.

Theoretically, heparin anticoagulation would terminate intravascular fibrin formation and permit replacement of platelets and clotting factors, but in practice this rarely succeeds more quickly than simple treatment of the septicaemia. It is only indicated if DIC and bleeding persist in spite of other treatment.

Complications of septicaemia and bacteraemia
One of the most common complications is that of metastatic infection. The most vascular tissues are most susceptible to bloodborne infection. In some instances infection reaches a tissue without any evidence of bacteraemia, as when osteomyelitis occurs in the growing bones of children.

Abscess formation.   Some organisms are particularly likely to produce abscesses. *Staph. aureus* can cause abscesses in skin, bone, breast, lung and other tissues. *Strep. milleri* especially causes brain and liver abscesses and is found in the majority of such lesions, sometimes associated with septicaemia or meningitis and sometimes not. Renal abscesses can follow bacteraemia due to Gram-negative bacilli.

Osteomyelitis.   *Staph. aureus* is by far the commonest pathogen of bone (Fig. 17) though in the Americas *H. influenzae* is also frequently recognized. *Salmonella spp.* can cause osteomyelitis in patients with sickle-cell disease, and bone infection is a recognized complication of enteric fever even in normal individuals. Positive blood cultures are by no means the rule in cases of osteomyelitis and aspiration of the bone lesions, or pus culture, may be necessary for diagnosis.

Meningitis.   Some pathogens, such as the meningococcus and pneumococcus, often produce meningitis together with septicaemia (possibly because they naturally exist in sites near the brain, but this is only speculation). Any septicaemia, however, can be associated with meningitis, and antibiotic therapy may then have to be modified to take account of the special problems of providing adequate doses to the meninges.

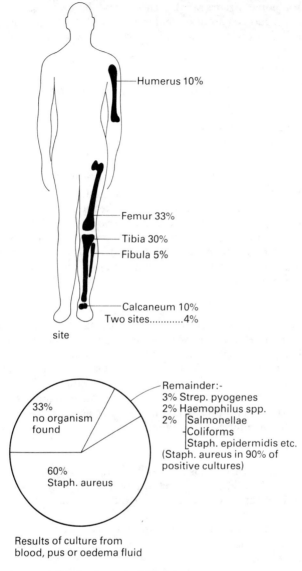

Fig. 17.   Osteomyelitis in the United Kingdom.

Endocarditis.   This is a danger in any septicaemia, even in patients with apparently normal heart valves. Fibrin thrombi in DIC or small emboli in intravenous drug abusers are recognized predisposing factors. The aortic and mitral valves are most commonly affected, but tricuspid valve disease sometimes occurs in intravenous drug abusers. Large vegetations are common and can produce loud murmurs. If the endocarditis cannot be controlled, gross breakdown of a valve may occur, and serious heart failure result.

Septicaemias due to Gram-positive cocci

Staphylococcal septicaemia

Epidemiology
Staphylococcus aureus is a resident of the skin and nares. It can enter the bloodstream via small skin injuries, infected lymph nodes, or from boils and carbuncles. Septicaemia can occur apparently spontaneously, often in young adults. It can also complicate chickenpox and severe influenza. It is the commonest septicaemia of intravenous drug abusers, who frequently have one or more subcutaneous abscesses at injection sites.

Patients with exfoliative dermatitis, epidermolysis or extensive infected eczema are at great risk of staphylococcal septicaemia which may be a terminal event.

Clinical features
Specific clinical features are few, so a searching history of predisposing factors should be obtained. Some patients have obvious staphylococcal skin lesions, or a rash of impetigo or small boils, but many do not. Rarely, a scarlatiniform rash like that of toxic shock syndrome occurs. A few patients have very severe pain on touching or moving their joints, a very helpful sign if it is present. Others may present with complications of septicaemia: staphylococcal pneumonia or lung abscess, osteomyelitis or occasionally meningitis.

Diagnosis
The total white cell count is misleading in the early stages, as it is often below 10×10^9/l, but a differential count will reveal 90% or more of neutrophils. After a number of days the total white cell count may rise to 14×10^9/l or more.

Blood cultures are almost always positive, and the organism can often be identified within 24 hours, so that bacteriological diagnosis is rarely a problem.

Treatment
Some *Staph. aureus* strains are sensitive to benzylpenicillin and can be eradicated by it.

The penicillinase-resistant penicillins remain the usual drugs of choice for penicillinase-producing *Staph. aureus* because they can be given in extremely high dosage, to provide high tissue levels with minimum toxicity. Cloxacillin and flucloxacillin are both penicillinase-resistant, and there is little to choose between them. Unfortunately a few staphylococci, mostly hospital-derived, or originating from Arabian countries, have developed resistance to these and many other drugs. This is not a common problem, but should be borne in mind when the response to treatment is unsatisfactory.

The narrow-spectrum cephalosporins including cephaloridine, cephradine and cephalothin are active against penicillinase-producing staphylococci, and cefuroxime can also be used, but the very wide-spectrum cefotaxime is not so effective.

Fusidic acid is an excellent antistaphylococcal agent which is well absorbed by mouth and need not always be given parenterally. If it is given alone, however, staphylococci quickly become resistant to it. It may be given in combination with any other antistaphylococcal agent.

From the range of aminoglycosides lincomycin is particularly valuable because of its good penetration of bones and soft tissues.

Most physicians like to use a penicillin in combination with fusidic acid or lincomycin, and to continue vigorous therapy for 10–14 days. Large abscesses should be aspirated or surgically drained. More prolonged treatment, often up to several weeks, is required if endocarditis or osteomyelitis occur. Lincomycin and fusidic acid both penetrate bone well, and make a useful combination for the treatment of osteomyelitis.

Streptococcus pyogenes septicaemia

Epidemiology
This infection is acquired by contamination of a wound by beta-haemolytic, Lancefield group A streptococci from the skin. Small cuts may become infected from surrounding skin, or organisms may be inoculated from another person's skin or infected site. This is a hazard to medical and nursing personnel.

In puerperal (childbed) fever the organism is introduced on instruments or the midwife's hands and enters via the placental bed. Finally, in a few cases, the streptococci spread from a focal infection in the throat or skin.

Clinical features
The wound at the site of entry may be trivial, and heal before septicaemia is established. Local evidence of infection can then be minimal, though pain or palpable swelling in local lymph nodes is a helpful sign of spread of infection. In a few cases, tissue necrosis occurs in and around the nodes. Sometimes 3 or 4 days elapse before severe illness is suspected.

The septicaemic illness appears rapidly, often with severe non-specific symptoms such as vomiting or diarrhoea, and can run its course in a matter of hours. Signs of pneumonia, peritonitis or meningitis may develop very quickly. Some patients have a scarlatiniform or erysipelas-like rash which aids diagnosis. In the most severe cases there is little opportunity for diagnositic investigation, while in others the space of a few days is afforded.

Diagnosis
A history of any predisposing factor is important in suggesting the diagnosis.

The white blood cell count is elevated, though not always above 13–14 $\times$ 10⁹/l, and shows a neutrophil leukocytosis. The total count may fall below 10 $\times$ 10⁹/l in late disease.

Blood cultures are usually positive, and the organism is quickly identifiable. Serological tests are rarely completed quickly enough to be of value.

Treatment
Strep. pyogenes is always sensitive to benzylpenicillin, which is the drug of choice. Cephalosporins such as cephradine and cephalothin, or erythromycin, are suitable alternatives. Treatment should be continued for 7–10 days in high dosage.

Poststreptococcal conditions, including nephritis, can complicate *Strep. pyogenes* septicaemia and may confuse the clinical picture by causing rashes, proteinuria or haematuria.

Other streptococcal septicaemias and bacteraemias

Pneumococcal infection
Pneumococcal infection is discussed more fully in the sections dealing with pneumonia and meningitis. Pneumococcal septicaemia occurs, though less commonly, in some other circumstances. Children of both sexes can suffer from primary pneumococcal peritonitis; in girls it is often associated with vaginitis and the organism can be isolated from vaginal swabs. Adult women can develop pelvic infection and septicaemia after childbirth or abortion. Recent splenectomy predisposes to pneumococcal septicaemia which can therefore attack those who have undergone splenectomy for congenital haemoglobinopathies, reticuloses or abdominal trauma. This predisposition diminishes over a number of years. Alcoholic cirrhosis also predisposes to pneumococcal infection, particularly peritonitis.

Pneumococci are almost always sensitive to penicillins, so that treatment is the same as for *Strep. pyogenes* infection. It should be continued for 14 days, however, because of a greater tendency to abscess formation, especially in intra-abdominal infection.

Microaerophilic streptococcal infections
These streptococci are found in the sinuses, the mouth and the genital tract. They tend to be untypable or sometimes of Lancefield group F. They can cause disease in all age groups and are particularly likely to be

associated with abscess formation. One of the group, *Strep. milleri* is the commonest organism isolated from both cerebral and hepatic abscesses and is also recognized as a cause of endocarditis, meningitis and septicaemia.

Although these infections are unusual, they are potentially treatable when recognized, as the streptococci are usually sensitive to penicillin.

Septicaemias due to Gram-negative cocci

Meningococcal septicaemia

This is similar in all respects, excepting meningeal involvement, to meningococcal meningitis, which is the commoner disease. Severe illness with rapid onset and the typical petechial or ecchymotic rash is associated with neutrophil leukocytosis, positive blood cultures and evidence of DIC. The CSF is normal. The course may be fulminating with bilateral adrenal haemorrhage (Waterhouse–Friderichsen syndrome) and death.

Treatment is the same as for meningitis, benzylpenicillin being the drug of choice.

Chronic meningococcal septicaemia
This is an unusual condition in which there is swinging fever, rash and arthritis, all of which wax and wane in cycles of several days. The rash is often macular or maculopapular, but may contain petechiae and small necrotic patches. Blood cultures are positive.

Treatment is the same as for acute meningococcal septicaemia. It should not be neglected as endocarditis, meningitis or acute septicaemia can occur at any stage of the illness.

Gonococcal septicaemia

Epidemiology
Septicaemia or complications of gonococcal bacteraemia are seen from time to time whenever gonorrhoea occurs. No predisposing factors are recognized, for septicaemia can occur in patients of either sex with uncomplicated or complicated disease.

Clinical features
The common features are those of a feverish illness with a rash. About half of women have a vaginal discharge or pelvic tenderness while a small proportion of men have unilateral epididymitis. The usual skin lesion is a tense painful vesicle often in the finger pulp or on the dorsum of the hand. When single, these lesions are difficult to distinguish from herpes simplex. Less commonly, multiple lesions are seen with a tendency to

haemorrhage, and occasionally a typical 'meningococcal' rash occurs.

Arthritis is common, affecting large joints, particularly the knee, wrist or ankle in which large effusions may occur.

Endocarditis is also seen, sometimes affecting the tricuspid valve, but more often on the left side of the heart.

In rare cases, perihepatic sepsis causes severe upper abdominal pain.

Diagnosis
There is a mild neutrophil leukocytosis. Blood cultures are often positive. Culture of synovial fluid tends to be negative until the later stages of illness, and this can cause difficulty in diagnosis.

In cases of doubt, urethral, rectal and cervical swabs may be positive. Culture of prostatic fluid obtained by massage can give a diagnosis in men when all else fails.

Caution.   Always carry out serological tests for syphilis, which coexists in 2 or 3% of cases of gonorrhoea.

Treatment
Benzylpenicillin is active against the majority of gonococci. Increasing numbers of penicillin-resistant strains are now seen, however, and the majority of these produce penicillinase. Cefuroxime has been found effective against penicillin-resistant strains and is also a useful drug in penicillin-sensitive patients.

Spectinomycin, used for uncomplicated gonorrhoea due to penicillin-resistant organisms, is only suitable for single intramuscular injection and may not be satisfactory when longer-term treatment is necessary.

Treatment is usually continued for 7–10 days, but longer courses may be needed if endocarditis or septic arthritis exists.

Septicaemias due to Gram-negative rods

Epidemiology
These organisms exist naturally in the small and large bowel, and frequently cause intra-abdominal and urinary tract infections. In young people, septicaemia can follow perforation of a peptic ulcer, gangrenous appendicitis, acute pancreatitis, pyelonephritis and abortion. About 20% of cases follow surgery or instrumentation.

In middle age, pyelonephritis, cholecystitis and abdominal or pelvic surgery are common predispositions, while in the elderly, urinary tract obstruction and abdominopelvic malignancies are important. There is a history of major surgery or of bladder instrumentation in 25–40% of elderly cases.

Escherichia coli is the most common cause of Gram-negative septicaemia; *Klebsiella spp* is sometimes seen. *Bacteroides fragilis* and other

Bacteroides spp are anaerobic Gram-negative rods derived from the colon or the female genital tract. They are quite common pathogens, and can exist in mixed infections.

Septicaemia with the multiply-resistant *Klebsiella* and *Pseudomonas spp.* occurs most often in patients with predisposition to Gram-negative infections who have received wide-spectrum antibiotics, and in patients with immune deficiencies.

Clinical features
The picture is typically that of a feverish patient with low or undetectable blood pressure. Any or all of the features of endotoxaemia may be present. A predisposing factor is often evident, but may not be.

Pseudomonas septicaemia is occasionally associated with the appearance of purple ulcerated skin lesions with erythematous borders (ecthyma gangrenosum).

Diagnosis
The white blood cell count may be raised but is not always, indeed it can be depressed in severe infections because of toxic effects on blood cells and bone marrow.

Blood culture will provide the definitive diagnosis. Cultures of urine, faeces or pus may be helpful

Gas–liquid chromatography (GLC) of pus or serum can demonstrate lipid fragments from anaerobic organisms.

Treatment
This should be commenced while resuscitation and microbiological assessment are carried out. It is usual to give a combination of drugs initially. For aerobic organisms gentamicin, other aminoglycosides, mezlocillin or cefotaxime may be used. Metronidazole is usually added to combat anaerobic pathogens (clindamycin is also active against anaerobes, but may predispose to pseudomembranous colitis). Cefoxitin is active against *B. fragilis*. Amikacin, ticarcillin, carbenicillin and azlocillin are useful agents against *Pseudomonas spp* and other highly resistant organisms.

Antibiotic therapy can be altered if necessary when culture and sensitivity results are available. In difficult cases the microbiologist may be able to suggest synergistic combinations of drugs, and to monitor serum levels of various agents. Gentamicin levels should always be monitored, as renal and cochlear damage occur easily in overdosage.

Complications
Reported complications of Gram-negative septicaemia and bacteraemia include abscesses, osteomyelitis, endarteritis, endocarditis and chest infections.

Unusual septicaemias

Gram-positive rods
Listeria monocytogenes (found in the genital tract, vegetable matter and in sewage) and *Erysipelothrix rhusiopathiae* (found in fish, shellfish, animals and meat) are unusual causes of septicaemia and of endocarditis. Affected patients are often, though not always, debilitated. If the organism is recovered from blood cultures, it may be dismissed as a 'contaminating diphtheroid' unless the microbiologist or the clinician has a suspicion of the diagnosis.

Fungal septicaemias
These are rare, and mainly confined to severely debilitated or immunodeficient patients. The degree of fever and leukocytosis is variable but the clinical picture of severe illness with multiple septic emboli and renal impairment is helpful. Fungal blood cultures should be set up to confirm the diagnosis. Treatment is with amphotericin or amphotericin plus flucytosine (which is active against yeasts), but the prognosis is often poor.

Drugs mentioned in this chapter

Drug	Indication	Usage and precautions
Amikacin	Gram-negative infections resistant to gentamicin	Dose for all ages is 15 mg/kg in two divided doses by intramuscular or intravenous injection; check blood levels; overdosage causes renal and cochlear damage
Amphotericin	Fungal infections	Starting dose 0.25 mg/kg daily by slow intravenous infusion, increasing by small aliquots to 0.5–1.0 mg/kg daily or alternate days; dose is limited by reactions including nausea, shock, rashes and rising blood urea; total dose given during course is usually 2.0–3.0 g
Azlocillin	Gram-negative infections, especially *Pseudomonas*	Adult dose 5.0 g 8-hourly by intravenous infusion; child's dose is a quarter to half of adult dose
Benzylpenicillin	Streptococcal, gonococcal and meningococcal infections;	Adult dose 2.4–3.0 g (4.0–5.0 mega units) 4 to 6-hourly intravenously by infusion (may be halved when patient is improv-

		sensitive *Staph. aureus* infections	ing); child's dose is a quarter to half of adult dose
Cefotaxime		Gram-negative and some *Pseudomonas* infections	Adult dose 2.0–3.0 g 6–8 hourly, intravenously; child's dose 150–200 mg/kg daily in two to four divided doses
Cefoxitin		Gram-negative and some *Bacteroides* infections	Adult dose 2.0 g 8-hourly intravenously; child's dose 80–160 mg/kg daily in divided doses
Cefsulodin		Narrow-spectrum anti-*pseudomonas*	
Cefuroxime		Gram-positive, *H. influenzae* and occasional coliform infections	Adult dose 1.5–3.0 g 6–8-hourly intravenously; child's dose 30–100 mg/kg daily in divided doses
Cephradine or cephalothin		Gram-positive infections; alternative to benzylpenicillin	Adult dose 1.0–1.5 g 4-hourly intravenously; child's dose 25 mg/kg 6-hourly
Dopamine		Falling blood pressure and cardiac output	Should not be used until volume replacement has raised venous pressure to normal; a solution of 800 μg/ml is made by dissolving 400 mg (two ampoules) in 500 ml of dextrose or saline solution, and infused at 5–20 μg/min (8 to 30 drops/min from a standard administration set); dose is adjusted according to response
Erythromycin		Alternative to penicillin in streptococcal infection	Adult dose 300–500 mg 6-hourly intravenously; child's dose 30–50 mg/kg daily in divided doses
Flucloxacillin or cloxacillin		Penicillinase-producing staphylococci	Adult dose 1.0–2.0 g 6-hourly intravenously; child's dose is a quarter to half of adult dose
Flucytosine		In combination with amphotericin for sensitive yeast infections	Dose for all ages 150–200 mg/kg daily, orally or intravenously; check blood count, as bone marrow depression occasionally occurs

Fusidic acid	Staphylococcal infections	Always used in combination; adult dose 500 mg 6-hourly or 1.0 g 8-hourly orally (may be given intravenously but readily causes phlebitis); child's dose 6–7 mg/kg 8-hourly
Gentamicin	Gram-negative infections (may be added to benzylpenicillin in group B streptococcal infections	Adult dose 60–120 mg 8-hourly by intramuscular or bolus intravenous injection, depending on peak and trough blood levels; ideal peak level 7–10 μg/ml; ideal trough level less than 2 μg/ml; peak level is estimated 1 hour after intramuscular or 15 minutes after intravenous injection; child's dose 6 mg/kg daily, in two divided doses for neonates and three divided doses for others
Hydrocortisone	Shock	Adult dose 500 mg to 1.0 g intravenously, may be repeated 6-hourly; child's dose 50–200 mg
Methylprednisolone	Shock	Sodium succinate (*not* acetate); adult dose 500 mg to 2.0 g by intravenous infusion in 10 to 20 minutes (not recommended while the CVP is low)
Latamoxef	Wide-spectrum including anaerobes	Adult dose 3.0–12.0 g daily in three 8-hourly doses by intramuscular or intravenous injection; child's dose 50 mg/kg 12-hourly; infant age 1–4 weeks 25 mg/kg 8-hourly; infant up to age 1 week 25 mg/kg 8-hourly
Lincomycin	Staphylococcal infections, including penicillin-resistant	Adult dose 600 mg by intramuscular injection once or twice daily *or* 600 mg by intravenous infusion 8–12-hourly; occasionally associated with pseudo-membranous colitis
Metronidazole	Anaerobic infections	Adult dose 500 mg 8-hourly by intravenous infusion, or 1.0 g 8-hourly, rectally (rectal dose 1.0 g 12-hourly after first 3 days); child's dose 7.5 mg/kg 8-hourly

		by any route; usual course is 7 days
Mezlocillin	Gram-negative infections, including *Pseudomonas*	Adult dose 5.0 g 6–8-hourly by intravenous infusion
Nitroprusside sodium	Endotoxic shock with severe acidosis	Ampoules of 50 mg are available; they may be dissolved in 500 ml or 1 l of intravenous infusion solution, giving concentrations of 100 or 50 μg/ml; infusion is started at 10–15 μg/min; up to 200 μg/min may be given to an adult
Ticarcillin	*Proteus* and *Pseudomonas* infections	Adult dose 15–20 g daily by rapid intravenous infusion, in divided doses
Tobramycin	Gram-negative infection resistant to gentamicin	Adult dose 3.0–5.0 mg/kg daily in three divided doses, by intramuscular or intravenous injection, or intravenous infusion; as with other aminoglycosides dose depends on blood levels (see gentamicin) and overdosage causes renal and cochlear damage; child's dose: up to age 1 week 2.0 mg/kg 12-hourly, older children 2.0–2.5 mg/kg 8-hourly

11

Clostridial and Related Infections

Introduction
The clostridia are Gram-positive, spore-forming, obligate anaerobes which are widely distributed in soil, and in the anaerobic environment of the colon of animals, and sometimes man. Diseases associated with *Clostridium botulinum* and *C. difficile* toxins have already been discussed in Chapter 5 (enteric infections and food poisoning). This chapter is concerned with the effects of clostridial invasion of tissues and of clostridial toxaemia.

Gas gangrene and related infections

Epidemiology
These infections result from the invasion of wounds by anaerobic organisms which can produce gas. The infecting pathogens are derived from animal or human faeces, or from soil. *C. perfringens* is the important pathogen in the majority of cases, but up to one-third of all cases may be caused by other clostridia (such as *C. septicum* or *C. bifermentans*), by anaerobic streptococci, or occasionally by *Escherichia coli* (which is a facultative anaerobe). Mixed infections are also seen, often derived from human faecal flora.

Chance contamination of wounds with clostridia is extremely common, but true infection can only develop when the environment favours anaerobic metabolism. Ischaemia is a major predisposing factor, so that the commonest type of gas gangrene seen in civilian practice involves the amputation stumps of arteriosclerotic limbs, or necrotic lesions on the lower limbs of arteriosclerotic or diabetic patients. On rare occasions the abdominal wall becomes infected after bowel surgery. Trauma, involving heavy soiling of wounds or much tissue death, is another predisposition which is much more common in times of war.

Apparently spontaneous gangrene may be associated with large-bowel perforation or malignancy.

Clinical features
These anaerobic infections can present in any of four distinct ways, each with a different prognosis.

Localized disease. In this case infection occurs only in a limited ischaemic area, such as a diabetic ulcer, a gangrenous toe or a small wound. Pain in the infected area is a strong indication of anaerobic infection. There is necrosis of the affected tissue and gas formation may or may not be detectable by eliciting local crepitus. A sweet-, acid-smelling serous discharge may be evident. Systemic upset and signs of toxaemia are rarely evident in such limited infection.

'Clostridial' cellulitis. This is a rapidly extending infection which affects the skin, subcutaneous tissue and fascial planes. It may occur anything from 2 days to 2 weeks or more after initial contamination. Pain in the affected area heralds the rapid appearance of subcutaneous oedema and large skin blisters which discharge the sweet-smelling serous fluid. Mauve discoloration of the skin, and serosanguineous discharge are sometimes seen. Gas formation is often obvious, with gross crepitus and gas in the skin blisters. The infection rarely spreads to normal muscle tissue.

Mild to moderate toxaemia is usually present, and results in haemolysis, reduced blood pressure, and rising blood urea and creatinine levels.

Clostridial myonecrosis. This is a severe, destructive infection of both muscle and the surrounding tissue. About 80% of cases are due to *C. perfringens*. Like cellulitis, it can begin days or weeks after the original injury, but gas formation may be slight in early cases. The patient develops fever, and severe pain in the affected site. The skin rapidly becomes mottled pale and purple, and haemorrhagic blisters appear. Gross oedema, affecting all tissues, produces huge enlargement of the limb. If muscle is exposed by incision, its surface appears pale grey and oedematous, while the interior is dark red and necrotic. The exudate has the characteristic sickly smell.

Toxaemia is severe. Haemolysis can occur very suddenly, reducing the haemoglobin level by several grams and producing jaundice, haemoglobinuria and acute renal tubular damage. The blood pressure may be barely recordable, and renal failure soon follows. In spite of profound shock, the patient is fully alert until the immediate preterminal stage.

Clostridial uterine infection. This is a special group among clostridial infections, as it is almost exclusively a sequel to septic abortion, usually illicitly procured. On rare occasions it follows normal delivery or gynaecological surgery.

Severe pelvic and back pain, offensive haemorrhagic discharge, fever and profound toxaemia make this one of the most severe types of clostridial infection. Death from shock, anaemia or renal failure can occur very early. Clostridial septicaemia is a frequent finding. Gas formation may not be evident clinically, unless the infection has spread to the perineum or abdominal wall. The cervix, uterus and fornices are oedematous and tender, and occasionally signs of uterine perforation are found.

Diagnosis
Blood examination.   There is a marked neutrophil leukocytosis which may reach $40 \times 10^9/l$ or more in severe cases. In severe toxaemia the red cell and platelet count are both low, and red cell fragments are seen in the blood film, indicating severe haemolysis.

The patient's blood group should be determined. Cross-matched blood may be required.

Urine examination.   Proteinuria is common. Haemoglobinuria occurs in severe haemolysis. Granular casts often appear in the urine of severe cases. A fall in the volume and specific gravity of the urine will give early warning of renal failure.

Microbiological investigation.   Wound exudate, blood cultures and excised tissue should be submitted for microscopy and culture. Evacuated uterine contents should also be examined.

Microscopy of the exudate often shows large numbers of Gram-positive bacilli, but a surprising lack of inflammatory cells. Culture in anaerobic conditions will confirm the identity of the pathogen.

Previous antibiotic treatment tends to make culture of the organism impossible in some cases. The clinical features, however, are often sufficiently characteristic to permit a correct diagnosis on these grounds alone.

X-ray examination.   This can reveal the presence of gas which is undetectable by clinical examination, and is also useful in demonstrating the extent of gas formation in the tissues.

Other investigations.   Estimation of haptoglobin or methaemalbumin levels can give a useful index of the extent of haemolysis at the time of initial assessment.

Apart from an unconjugated hyperbilirubinaemia due to haemolysis, there is often a mild or moderate hepatocellular disturbance of the liver function tests caused by toxaemia.

Frequent estimation of the haemoglobin, creatinine and urea levels is necessary, as these can change quite suddenly in a toxaemic patient.

Treatment
Initial assessment and resuscitation.   Except in the localized type of infection this is of major importance. An intravenous infusion should be commenced while blood is drawn for initial investigation. In addition to

electrolyte solutions, plasma or plasma protein fraction are useful, and whole blood may be given if the patient is already anaemic. An infusion of mannitol may improve renal function if this does not respond adequately to volume replacement.

X-ray assessment can be made during arrangements for immediate treatment.

Antibiotics. The antibiotic of choice is benzylpenicillin which is active against both clostridia and many streptococci. Wider-spectrum drugs, such as aminoglycosides, cephalosporins or penicillins should be added if coliform or mixed infection is likely, as in abdominal wall infection. It is doubtful whether the antibiotic will penetrate already necrotic and ischaemic tissue, but it may inhibit the spread of infection to adjacent healthy tissue. High-dose intravenous therapy is therefore justified.

Antiserum. Anti-gas gangrene serum (AGGS) is not nowadays thought to be of use in combating infection.

Hyperbaric oxygen. This is strongly recommended by those who have access to it and is often used before emergency surgical treatment. After an initial treatment of about 90 minutes at 250 kPa (2½ atmospheres (atm)) there can be a distinct improvement in many patients with clostridial infection. Both toxaemia and tissue invasion are ameliorated. Non-clostridial infections do not respond well, however.

Treatment may be continued two or three times daily until there is clinical evidence of healing. The only limitation of treatment is the occurrence of convulsions due to oxygen toxicity, or of 'claustrophobia' in the high-pressure tank, in a small minority of patients.

Surgery. This is often essential. In localized infection, it can be restricted to simple excision of necrotic tissue or amputation of an affected toe. In cellulitis, widespread removal of affected tissue is necessary, and may need to be followed by revision and, after recovery, by skin grafting. In myonecrosis both skin and muscle must be removed, often by amputation of a limb or higher amputation of a stump. Fulminating disease may spread so rapidly as to defy surgery because of its enormous extent.

An infected uterus should be evacuated to remove infected tissue. In rare instances hysterectomy may be indicated in an attempt to terminate severe toxaemia.

Treatment with antibiotics, hyperbaric oxygen and supportive measures should be continued until gas formation ceases and healing is obviously in progress.

Prophylaxis
Adequate wound toilet, including removal of foreign matter and non-

viable tissue, should be carried out as soon as possible after injury. Early closure of soiled wounds should be avoided.

Prophylactic antibiotics are of value, and are widely used in military practice. Benzylpenicillin, given intramuscularly at operation for leg amputations, or as soon as possible after injury, is the drug of choice.

Tetanus

Epidemiology
Tetanus is a disease caused by tetanospasmin, a toxin of *Clostridium tetani*. This organism is plentiful in soil and horse manure. It exists in the bowel of horses and other herbivores, but not usually in man.

The usual means of infection is contamination of a wound with soil or manure. Farmers and rose-growers are therefore among those most at risk. In communities where contact with animal dung is usual, neonatal tetanus can follow infection of the umbilical stump. The neurotoxin is elaborated in anaerobic conditions, which are often found in deep lacerations or puncture wounds. The wound need not be serious, however, for up to one-third of patients cannot recall a recent injury.

On rare occasions a chronically infected middle ear is invaded by *C. tetani*.

Clinical features
The onset of tetanus can occur from a few days to 3 weeks, or more, after injury, but is usually between 7 and 14 days. An early onset indicates severe disease.

The effect of the toxin is to increase the excitability of motor neurones so that any movement or reflex activity causes powerful muscle contraction. In severe cases, autonomic motor function is also affected.

The earliest sign is the appearance of trismus (lockjaw), a contraction of the jaw muscles provoked by facial movement, swallowing or a startle. Sensitivity may progress to the pharyngeal muscles, the diaphragm and all of the skeletal muscles. Three main grades of severity are usually distinguished.

Mild.   There is late onset of trismus, but this does not become sufficiently severe to progress to dysphagia or respiratory embarrassment.

Moderate.   There is dysphagia and some interference with normal respirations. Fleeting spasms of generalized muscle contraction may occur.

Severe.   Apart from interference with swallowing and breathing, there are frequent generalized spasms of muscle contraction. The face is contorted into the 'risus sardonicus', the spine is arched into opisthotonos, the legs extended and the arms flexed. This results in severe, cramp-like pain. The rigid diaphragm and laryngeal spasm make respiration impossible. The strength of the spinal muscles is sufficient to cause crush fractures of vertebrae.

In the most severe cases, autonomic dysfunction causes extremes of tachycardia and bradycardia with proportional changes in the blood pressure.

The patient soon dies of respiratory failure, aspiration pneumonia, dysrrhythmia or exhaustion.

The usual duration of moderate to severe tetanus is 3 or 4 weeks, with approximately equal phases of worsening, static disease and improvement. Muscle stiffness may persist for several weeks after recovery.

Local tetanus. This occurs in partly immune patients and consists of stiffness or spasm near the site of injury. The mechanism of this is probably the local invasion of the spinal cord by toxin which has passed up the peripheral nerves. It does not usually progress to severe tetanus.

Cephalic tetanus. This is local tetanus of the cranial muscles adjacent to an infected middle ear. In some patients, whose facial nerve is damaged as it passes through the infected ear, there is spasm only on the normal side of the face.

Diagnosis

Not all wound infections with *C. tetani* lead to tetanus, indeed, some of the organisms are non-toxigenic. A positive wound smear or culture in the absence of clinical evidence is *not* diagnostic, it only confirms the possibility of the diagnosis. In addition to this, there are no characteristic laboratory findings in tetanus. The diagnosis is therefore clinical. Early suspicion is necessary if prompt treatment is to be given, and care must be taken not to dismiss the initial symptoms as hysterical.

Treatment

All patients should have an intravenous cannula in place, so that muscle spasm can be treated promptly. Intravenous benzylpenicillin is given for the first 7 days, to eradicate the clostridia. Nursing in a quiet, dark room will help to avoid excess stimulation of reflex muscle activity. Adequate analgesia must be provided for muscle pain.

Human tetanus immune globulin (HTIG). This is given intramuscularly in a dose of 30–300 units/kg, depending on the severity at presentation.

Mild cases. Sedation is essential, and diazepam is valuable for this as it has a muscle relaxant action and helps to ameliorate trismus. Most patients can take a soft diet but, if trismus prevents this, nasogastric feeding is necessary.

Moderate cases. These patients require nasogastric feeding, and tracheostomy to avoid the effects of laryngeal spasm. As generalized muscle spasms are slight, they can be allayed by heavy sedation. Care must be taken in the use of diazepam as, once it has saturated the body fat, it is excreted slowly, with a half-life of about 48 hours. Prolonged high dosage may therefore be cumulative.

Severe cases. Sedation is insufficient in these cases to suppress generalized muscle spasms, so complete neuromuscular blockade must be induced and artificial ventilation carried out. Beta-blockade may be necessary to alleviate extreme tachycardia. Chest and urinary infections commonly occur, and can be treated with antibiotics given either via the nasogastric tube or intramuscularly. Regular subcutaneous heparin may reduce the chance of venous thrombosis during paralysis.

Muscle relaxants can be discontinued gradually and replaced by sedation as the motor excitability diminishes.

The overall mortality rate is less than 10% in western countries.

Prophylaxis
Active immunization with tetanus toxoid is offered to all infants in the United Kingdom. Booster immunization every 10 years is sufficient to maintain immunity. Farmers and others are urged to accept immunization, as *an attack of tetanus confers no immunity.*

At the time of injury. Wound toilet, as for prevention of gas gangrene, is most important.

If the patient is previously immunized, a booster dose of tetanus toxoid should be given.

If the patient is unimmunized, or the immune status is unknown, the first dose of tetanus toxoid should be given immediately, and human tetanus immunoglobulin (HTIG) 250 units given intramuscularly at a different site. The two remaining doses of tetanus toxoid must be given later, according to the usual schedule.

Drugs mentioned in this chapter

Drug	Indication	Usage and precautions
Benzylpenicillin	Eradication of clostridia from wounds	Adult dose 1.2–2.4 g (2–4 mega units) 4–6-hourly, intravenously; child's dose is a quarter to half of adult dose
Cephalothin or cephradine	Alternative to penicillin	Adult dose 1.0–1.5 g 4-hourly intravenously; child's dose 25 mg/kg 6-hourly

Gentamicin	*Escherichia coli* and other entero-bacteriaceae	Adult dose 60–120 mg 8-hourly by intramuscular or bolus intravenous injection; dose depends on peak and trough blood levels (see Chapter 10); child's dose 6.0 mg/kg daily in two divided doses for neonates and three doses for others
Metronidazole	Addition to other drugs, useful in mixed anaerobic infections	Adult dose 500 mg 8-hourly by intravenous infusion or 1.0 g 8-hourly rectally (rectal dose reduced to 500 mg 8-hourly after 3 days); child's dose 7.5 mg/kg 8-hourly by either route
Tetanus toxoid (Tet/Vac/Ads)	Active immunization against tetanus	Adult primary immunization: 0.5 ml by intramuscular or deep subcutaneous injection; three doses are given, the interval between the first two doses should be 6–8 weeks, the third dose is given 6 months after the second Booster doses may be given at 5–10-year intervals; more frequent dosage increases the likelihood of hypersensitivity reactions

12

Infective Endocarditis

Introduction
Endocarditis is inflammation of the interior of the heart. Infection tends
to occur in areas where the lining of the heart is made 'sticky' by adherent
platelet thrombi, and micro-organisms become attached. The laminar
flow of blood normally prevents aggregation of platelets at the vessel wall
but, where turbulence is great, there are stagnant areas among the eddies
where platelets can alight. Further layers of thrombus protect the
attached micro-organisms from the bacteriocidal action of the blood.

Typically, infective endocarditis occurs on the low-pressure side of a
small orifice, in mitral and aortic stenosis and on small ventricular septal
defects. Other areas affected include patent ductus arteriosus, coarc-
tation of the aorta, and mural thrombus after myocardial infarction.

Although rheumatic heart disease has long been regarded as the major
precursor of infective endocarditis, it is now equalled by congenital disorders, and acquired conditions related to ischaemic heart disease or
collagen diseases.

'Spontaneous' endocarditis.   About half of these infections occur on
valves known to be damaged previously. The commonest causative
organism is *Streptococcus viridans* which is derived from the oral flora. A
minority of patients have a recent history of dental manipulation. About
one-tenth of cases are due to faecal streptococci derived from the urinary
or genital tract and the bowel. Catheterization, urethroscopy and inser-
tion of intrauterine contraceptive devices have been followed by this type
of infection. Elderly patients may have infections due to diphtheroids,
coliforms and other Gram-positive and Gram-negative organisms.

Postsurgical endocarditis.   Patients are at risk of endocarditis for up to 3
months after open heart surgery. The organism most often responsible is
Staphylococcus epidermidis. Late cases may be due to fungal infection,
particularly with *Candida spp.*

Endocarditis in intravenous drug abusers.   In Great Britain this is almost
always due to *Staph. aureus*, and patients often have staphylococcal skin
abscesses. In the United States a number of other bacteria are found,
including *Serratia spp.* and mixed Gram-positive and Gram-negative
infection.

The tricuspid valve may be the site of infection in this group of patients.

Culture-negative endocarditis.   This group includes patients in whom culture has been made impossible by antibiotic treatment or by extreme fastidiousness of their organisms. Part of this group, however, suffer from infection with *Coxiella burnetii, Chlamydia psittaci* or fungal pathogens.

Clinical features
Early features.   Most cases have an extremely insidious onset with fever, malaise and night sweats. There is almost always a heart murmur but it may change its character very little at this stage. After a variable number of days or weeks the erythrocyte sedimentation rate (ESR) rises, the patient loses weight and clubbing of the fingers appears.

Features of progressive tissue damage.   After a period of several days or weeks large vegetations form on the affected valve. Fragments of these vegetations periodically break off, causing embolic episodes and progressively damaging the valve. The emboli can cause small infarcts in the kidney, bowel and skin, or larger and more serious obstructions of limb arteries or cerebral arteries. Multiple pulmonary emboli can occur in right-sided endocarditis. Sometimes these embolic phenomena are the presenting features of the disease.

It is at this stage that the cardiac murmur changes, as vegetations form and break. Very large vegetations may obstruct a valve, as sometimes happens in fungal endocarditis and this can result in sudden severe heart failure. Sudden disruption of valve cusps can also take place with similar gross haemodynamic effects. The importance of frequent examination of the patient at this stage cannot be overemphasized.

Late clinical features.   Eventually the immunological effects of prolonged infection result in further clinical features. Splenomegaly may be detectable. Vasculitis is common, with petechial rashes on the skin, conjunctivae and other mucous membranes, and with associated haematuria. Osler's nodes, small tender, necrotic swellings, appear on the skin. Roth's spots, the ocular counterpart of Osler's nodes, appear as pale, flame shapes with a red margin in the optic fundi. Immune complexes can cause nephritis, with protein and red-cell casts in the urine, and with deteriorating renal function.

Diagnosis
This depends on the degree of clinical suspicion and detection of changing clinical features in the patient. The rising ESR, finger clubbing and heart murmur are often the earliest recognized clinical features, but any persistent fever in a patient with known valvular heart disease should suggest endocarditis until proved otherwise.

Positive blood cultures are extremely important in both diagnosis and management. Because bacteraemia is intermittent, four to six separate blood cultures should be carried out before treatment. (In urgent cases they can be taken during a period of 1 hour.)

About one-fifth of patients have negative blood cultures. In these cases fungal blood cultures should be requested, and a serum sample should be taken for later estimation of *Coxiella* and *Chlamydia* antibodies in paired sera. Fungal infections can also be detected sometimes by serological methods.

Echocardiography can show vegetations on heart valves and is useful in demonstrating their disappearance with treatment. Negative echocardiographic results, however, do not always exclude the possibility of endocarditis.

Treatment
If endocarditis is suspected, treatment should be commenced as soon as initial blood cultures and serological samples have been collected. The chance of a fatal embolism or other complication increases with the duration of untreated disease.

'Spontaneous' endocarditis.   The majority of cases of this type can be treated with benzylpenicillin to which *Strep. viridans* is sensitive. Until the organism has been identified, however, it is desirable to add gentamicin to the regimen, as penicillin-resistant streptococci are occasionally responsible. An elderly patient, or one who has recently had urinary or genital tract manipulation, should always receive gentamicin initially.

Antibiotic levels of eight to ten times the minimum inhibitory concentration (MIC) for the organism are ideal, though they cannot always be achieved with the more toxic drugs. Bacteriocidal agents should always be used when possible. In a disease as serious as endocarditis, a vague history of being 'allergic' to penicillin should not exclude its use. Penicillin may be administered (with antianaphylaxis treatment readily available) unless there is a previous history of anaphylaxis. Alternatives to penicillin include cephradine and cefuroxime.

If penicillin-resistant streptococci are isolated, a combination of ampicillin and gentamicin may be more appropriate.

Postsurgical endocarditis and endocarditis in intravenous drug abusers. *Staph. epidermidis* and *Staph. aureus* are often resistant to benzylpenicillin. In infections where staphylococci may be present, a combination of cloxacillin or flucloxacillin with fusidic acid is the treatment of choice, as the penicillins can be given in very high doses and the fusidic acid has excellent tissue-penetrating properties. Benzylpenicillin and gentamicin can be substituted for cloxacillin if wider-spectrum treatment is desirable while the identification of the staphylococcus is confirmed.

Coxiella and Chlamydiae.   The recommended treatment for these is tetracycline, which may be given orally. If this cannot be tolerated, erythromycin is a useful alternative.

Duration of treatment
In all cases therapy should be continued for at least 4, and preferably for 6 weeks to ensure eradication of organisms buried in platelet thrombi. The need for further antibiotic treatment should be considered at the end of this time. (Erythromicin may be added to the last 2 weeks of penicillin therapy in case cell-wall-deficient organisms (L-forms) have emerged during treatment.)

Fungal endocarditis.   This is a relatively rare and serious problem. Amphotericin is the treatment of choice, to which flucytosine should be added if yeasts are present. Fungal infection cannot always be eradicated by medical treatment, even if the infected valve is removed, and long-term maintenance therapy may be necessary to prevent recrudescence of disease.

Place of surgery.   Valve replacement is an important part of management. In bacterial endocarditis, antibiotic treatment alone may be sufficient or, if it is not, a severely damaged valve can often be replaced after the infection has been controlled. In other types of endocarditis the available medical treatment is less satisfactory. Valve excision and replacement may be necessary to control the infection and, in fungal endocarditis to remove the risk of serious embolism.

If a left heart valve is suddenly destroyed, emergency replacement may be required to avert heart failure. In all cases it is an advantage to operate when blood levels of antibiotics are adequate.

Complications
Antibiotic hypersensitivity.   This can develop during a prolonged course of treatment. It can often be controlled with modest doses of corticosteroids and antihistamines but, if it is not, a change of antibiotic is indicated.

Abscess formation.   Abscesses can form in the valve-rings and septum of the heart, and sometimes penetrate the myocardium to produce a pericardial effusion. Emergency surgery is often required in such cases, and preoperative angiography can give a good indication of the site of the abscess.

Mycotic aneurisms.   Blood vessel walls are weakened in sites where septic emboli alight, and can rupture. Surgical intervention may be useful if massive haemorrhage occurs, but intracerebral haemorrhage is rarely amenable to this. The use of anticoagulants in patients with endocarditis is contraindicated because of this problem.

Renal failure.   This may occur as a result of glomerulonephritis, or in association with heart failure. It is treated in the standard way.

Heart failure.   This can be due to defective heart valves or to secondary myocarditis. Digoxin is valuable in treatment.

Mortality.   This varies between different reports. In developed countries it is 20–40%.

Prophylaxis
Many episodes of infective endocarditis can be avoided by preventing bacteraemia. Bacteraemia is usual during dental treatment, and common during instrumentation of the bladder, uterus, bowel and pancreas. It seems to be unusual during childbirth.
    Antibiotics are given, so as to achieve a maximum blood level at the anticipated time of the bacteraemia.

Recommended before dental treatment.   Amoxycillin 3.0 g orally one hour before treatment, *or* benzylpenicillin 600 mg intramuscularly 30 minutes before, 4 and 8 hours after, treatment.

Recommended for cystoscopy or genital instrumentation.   Ampicillin 1.0 g and gentamicin 80 mg intramuscularly 1 hour before procedure.

Recommended before cardiac surgery.   Fusidic acid 500 mg and gentamicin 80 mg intravenously during induction of anaesthesia.
    Treatment for longer periods before or after procedures is likely to change the body flora and result in bacteraemia due to resistant organisms.

Hazards of intravenous cannulation
An indwelling intravenous cannula offers open access for bacteria and fungi to pass from the skin to the circulation. In endocarditis this is particularly important, as any bacteraemia can give rise to new infection. The problem can be minimized by inserting cannulae with full aseptic precautions and by changing them every 2–3 days. Catheters inserted into central veins and buried in a small skin tunnel (Brody–Hickman cannulae) may be left in position for the duration of treatment because the venous puncture is far from the skin puncture.
    Thrombophlebitis and thrombus on the catheter can be minimized by

the addition of 500 units of heparin to each 500 ml of infusion fluid. Some physicians recommend weekly flushing of long-term cannulae with 10 mg amphotericin, to discourage overgrowth of fungi.

In a few units, each dose of antibiotic is given by a separate venepuncture, but this can be very distasteful and distressing for some patients.

Blood cultures should be repeated at intervals during therapy to ensure that further organisms have not appeared. The ESR should fall towards normal as infection is controlled.

Follow-up
Repeated physical examination in the weeks after recovery will ensure that new changes in the heart sounds, or the reappearance of finger clubbing and other signs do not go unnoticed. A new rise in the ESR may be an important early warning of relapse or reinfection.

Drugs mentioned in this chapter

The drugs used for the treatment of endocarditis are the same in general as those used for the treatment of septicaemia. In endocarditis the highest possible dose must usually be given for 4–6 weeks, and it is therefore important to use the least toxic drug possible, or a drug whose serum level is easily measured (see Chapter 10).

Additional drug information

Drug	Indication	Usage and precautions
Amoxycillin and probenecid (oral)	May be used for continuation therapy in sensitive *Strep. viridans* infections	Adult dose amoxycillin 500 mg to 1.0 g 6-hourly, orally *plus* probenecid 500 mg 9-hourly orally; child's dose: a quarter to a half of adult dose of amoxycillin *plus* probenecid 40 mg/kg daily in divided doses (children over 50 kg should take adult's doses); gastrointestinal disturbance can limit the use of this regimen
Erythromycin	Alternative to tetracycline in chlamydia and *Coxiella* infections	Adult doses: 300 to 500 mg 6-hourly intravenously or 1.0 g 6–8-hourly orally; child's doses 50 mg/kg daily intravenously or 250–500 mg 6-hourly orally
Tetracycline	Chlamydia and *Coxiella* infections	Oxytetracycline adult dose 750 mg 9-hourly orally; doxycycline 200 mg then 100–200 mg 12-

hourly orally (does not cause rising blood urea, as other tetracyclines can); tetracyclines cause damage to the growing teeth and bones of children

13

Tuberculosis

Epidemiology
Tuberculosis is a granulomatous disease due to infection with a mycobacterium. The great majority of cases are caused by *Mycobacterium tuberculosis*, and three-quarters of these cases have pulmonary tuberculosis. Any tissue of the body, however, can be affected by tuberculosis and a quarter of cases have non-pulmonary disease. A small percentage of cases have disease in more than one part of the body.

There are about 30 mycobacteria which cause granulomatous disease in man, but most of them are rare compared with *M. tuberculosis*. Those which are occasionally encountered are *M. bovis* (rare in western countries where bovine tuberculosis has been eradicated), *M. kansasii*, *M. xenopei* and mycobacteria of the avium-intracellulare group. The last three are found predominantly in patients with pre-existing chest disease, or abnormalities of cell-mediated immunity. Other mycobacteria, including *M. chelonei*, *M. fortuitum* and *M. marinum* tend to cause skin nodules and abscesses after accidental inoculation. *M. ulcerans* is a cause of tropical ulcers.

Various routes of infection are recognized in the transmission of tuberculosis.

Airborne transmission. This is probably by far the commonest means of spread, and is responsible for the infectious nature of 'open' pulmonary tuberculosis (in which mycobacteria are shed in the sputum).

Ingestion. This is important in the spread of *M. bovis* which heavily contaminates the milk of tuberculous cows. It can result in abdominal disease or glandular disease.

Haematogenous spread. This must be the means of infection of bones and the kidneys, as well as the origin of miliary tuberculosis. Those organs with the greatest blood supply are most often affected.

Inoculation. This is a common route of infection of the skin, either accidentally through scratches or therapeutic injection sites, or by autoinoculation from a pre-existing focus.

Susceptibility to tuberculosis depends on a wide variety of factors, of which a common one worldwide is the nutritional and social status of the community. Overcrowding combined with debility due to malnutrition increases the prevalence of tuberculosis in a community.

People of different races have different predispositions. Caucasians tend to develop pulmonary and renal disease, commoner in elderly men. Indian-Asian groups, however, are prone to glandular disease of adolescents and young adults, as well as pulmonary disease in all age-groups. Eskimos and North American Indians are susceptible to severe and disseminated disease.

Patients with defective cell-mediated immunity are particularly susceptible to pulmonary and disseminated tuberculosis. It is a recognized cause of fever in those with Hodgkin's disease and lymphatic leukaemias.

Clinical features of tuberculosis
Three different types of tuberculous infection are recognized; primary, disseminated and reactivated. Primary tuberculosis is the result of first acquisition of the organism, and is associated with the development of an immune response to tuberculoprotein. Disseminated disease follows haematogenous distribution of the organism from its site of entry, or from a focus of infection, to different parts of the body. Reactivated tuberculosis is disease occurring in a person who has previously developed an immune reaction to tuberculoprotein. This type of infection often results in extensive, destructive lesions.

Any type of the disease may exist without causing significant symptoms, but cases usually present with a typical quartet of fever, malaise, night sweats and weight loss. Additional local symptoms may indicate the site of infection. Few other conditions produce this picture but drug fevers, brucellosis, lymphoreticular malignancy, renal tumour and rare, persistent viral infections can cause similar symptoms.

Clinical features of primary tuberculosis (Fig. 18)
In primary tuberculosis a small focus of infection is quickly surrounded by an encapsulating granuloma, which tends to heal by fibrosis and later to calcify. The draining lymph nodes are often enlarged, and contain granulomata which heal in the same way.

Erythema nodosum.   This is sometimes an accompaniment of primary tuberculosis infection, particularly in children and young adults. Although it is also associated with several other conditions, it should always prompt the physician to investigate the possibility of tuberculosis.

Primary pulmonary tuberculosis.   The primary granuloma in the lung (Ghon focus) tends to appear in the periphery of the mid-zone. It is often accompanied by enlargement of the hilar lymph nodes on the same side, and these two lesions together constitute the primary complex (of

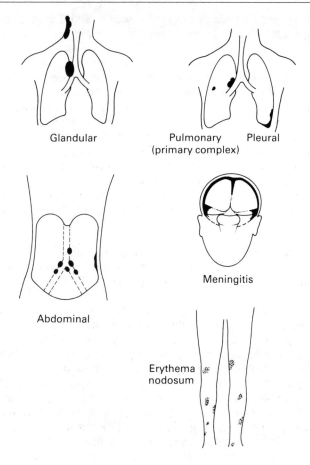

Glandular

Pulmonary
(primary complex)

Pleural

Abdominal

Meningitis

Erythema
nodosum

Fig. 18. Manifestations of primary tuberculosis.

Ranke). Apart from the typical quartet of symptoms, some patients have a cough because of bronchial irritation, or vague central chest pain due to hilar lymph node enlargement. It is likely that many infections are unrecognized, as a calcified primary lesion is a fairly common finding on routine chest X-ray.

Primary pleural tuberculosis. In this case the granulomatous lesion is in the pleura. The usual symptoms are accompanied by pleuritic pain, which may disappear as the two layers of pleura become separated by an effusion. A moderate-sized effusion will cause shortness of breath, but very small effusions are common, and these cause no symptoms. If an effusion is too small to cause a significant area of dullness to percussion

and reduced breathsounds, it can still be seen as an infilling of the cos-
tophrenic angle on chest X-ray. Large effusions are less often seen.

Tuberculous pericarditis.   Granulomata of the pericardium cause ret-
rosternal chest pain which is often pleuritic in nature, and which is less
severe in the erect than in the supine posture. The pain tends to become
dull as an effusion develops. Small effusions cause little haemodynamic
disturbance, and may only be detectable by echocardiography.

Large effusions cause shortness of breath and signs of cardiae tam-
ponade; the systemic blood pressure is low, the jugular venous pressure is
elevated and it rises further on inspiration, instead of falling as it does in
normal circumstances. Gross congestive heart failure is rarely seen. On
chest X-ray the heart shadow is large, pear-shaped and may show a double
outline. Healing by fibrosis can sometimes result in constrictive
pericarditis.

Primary tuberculous meningitis.   This has been discussed previously
(see Chapter 9). It is most common in children in whom it develops
usually in the first few months after exposure to infection.

Lymph node tuberculosis.   This is particularly common in young adults
of Asian origin, in whom it is the commonest non-respiratory presentation of tuberculosis. A lymph node, or group of nodes, become
increasingly swollen and the patient complains of typical symptoms of
tuberculosis. Cervical or mediastinal nodes are most often affected. Cervical lymph node enlargement is usually soon obvious, but swelling of
intrathoracic nodes may not be discovered until vague, central chest pain
leads to X-ray examination. Large intrathoracic nodes may press on
neighbouring bronchi, causing wheeze and shortness of breath. Total
bronchial occlusion causes collapse of the segment or lobe. The *middle
lobe syndrome* of children is collapse of the middle lobe due to pressure on
its bronchus when hilar lymph nodes enlarge.

On rare occasions an enlarged node may rupture into a large bronchus,
or even into the trachea, causing sudden respiratory obstruction, and
releasing mycobacteria into the bronchial tree.

Primary abdominal tuberculosis.   In this case the site of the granuloma
among the abdominal viscera may be impossible to detect, but enlargement and granuloma formation occurs in many abdominal lymph nodes.
Ascites collects insidiously and may become massive if neglected. Most
patients have abdominal discomfort or pain, and the majority have typical symptoms of tuberculosis.

Diagnosis of primary tuberculosis
Blood examination.   This is rarely helpful as there is no characteristic
change in the white cell count, which may be normal or slightly raised.

The ESR also may be slightly raised, up to 40 or 50 mm/hour, but in a few cases it remains normal. The ESR is very high when erythema nodosum occurs.

Slight elevation of aspartate transaminase or alkaline phosphatase levels is not unusual.

X-ray studies. The chest X-ray is of major diagnostic importance. In primary pulmonary tuberculosis, the appearance may be characteristic. A pleural or pericardial effusion will be well-demonstrated in most cases, and mediastinal lymph node enlargement may not be demonstrable by any other means. Wherever the suspected site of the lesion, a chest X-ray should be carried out, as almost a quarter of patients with non-pulmonary disease also have pulmonary lesions.

Bacteriology of sputum or effusion. Smears may be stained with Ziehl–Neelsen stain or with fluorescent auromine stain to demonstrate acid-fast bacteria, but in primary tuberculosis few organisms escape from the granuloma and staining may reveal none. Culture, similarly, is often negative but should be carried out, as it is diagnostic when positive.

Tuberculous effusions usually contain a modest number of lymphocytes and have a high protein level and a lowered glucose level. This helps to distinguish them from pyogenic or 'rheumatic' effusions, which often contain neutrophils.

Examination of biopsy specimens. This can be very helpful. In particular cervical lymph nodes and pleura can be biopsied easily. Abdominal lymph nodes are often accessible at laparoscopy. Not only is histological examination important in revealing granulomata or mycobacteria, but culture of the tissue is likely to be positive and allow determination of the organism's drug sensitivities.

The tuberculin test (Fig. 19). This test detects delayed hypersensitivity to tuberculoprotein (purified protein derivative or PPD).

In the *Mantoux test* 0.1 ml of PPD is injected intradermally into the flexor aspect of the forearm, and the resulting area of induration is measured 48–72 hours later. Induration of 6 mm, or more, diameter indicates a positive result while 15 mm or more is a 'strong positive'. Two dilutions of PPD are regularly used; people with acquired immunity or who have had BCG immunization have a positive response to 1:1000 PPD (total dose of 10 tuberculin units (TU)); those with active disease or regular contact with tuberculosis often have a strongly positive response to 1:10 000 PPD (total dose 1.0 TU), and may have a severe local reaction with blistering or ulceration to 1:1000 PPD. (1:100 PPD is used as a test of ability to mount a response in patients with poor immunity.)

The *Heaf test* is a screening tuberculin test widely used in Britain. Undiluted PPD is spread over about 1 cm diameter of skin and a 'Heaf

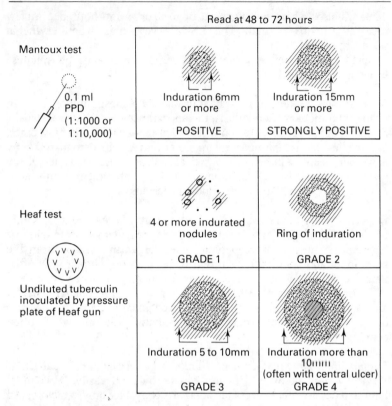

Fig. 19.   Tuberculin testing.

gun' is used to press eight tiny stylets through the PPD into the epidermis. The results are read at 48–72 hours and are expressed according to the reaction at some or all of the puncture sites.

The tuberculin test takes 4–6 weeks to convert from negative to positive when primary infection occurs. If it is negative, therefore, when tuberculosis is suspected, it should be repeated *at the same dilution* after an interval of about 3 weeks.

A conversion from negative to positive, a positive Mantoux test at 1:10 000 dilution, or a grade III or IV Heaf response indicate tuberculosis unless proved otherwise. False negative reactions occur in severe debility, during acute viral infections and in overwhelming tuberculous disease.

Disseminated tuberculosis

Disseminated tuberculosis results when mycobacteria are spread throughout the body by the bloodstream.

Miliary tuberculosis

In this form of tuberculosis, small granulomata are evenly distributed throughout the body. They are visible in the chest X-ray as even-sized nodules a millimetre or two in diameter (looking miliary, that is, like millet seeds). They can also be seen macroscopically and microscopically on liver biopsy. Occasionally, tubercles are visible as small white dots in the optic fundi.

The typical symptoms of tuberculosis are usually present. Vague chest and abdominal discomfort are not unusual. Debility, anaemia and hypoproteinaemia develop quickly in untreated cases.

Occult tuberculosis

This presentation is seen most often in Asian-Indian men, but can occur in any age-group and in any ethnic group. The patient quickly develops a high swinging fever, becomes sleepless and anorexic and loses weight rapidly. Night sweats are usual.

Apart from fever, there may be no abnormal physical findings at all, though sometimes a few lymph nodes are enlarged or the liver edge is palpable. In untreated cases the fever will continue unchanged for weeks or months.

Diagnosis of disseminated tuberculosis.

Blood examination. There is no typical change in the blood picture. Bone-marrow involvement may result in a low white blood cell count and anaemia; rarely a leukaemoid rise in the count occurs. The ESR is usually raised and is often above 70 mm/hour in occult tuberculosis.

Mild elevation of aspartate transaminase and alkaline phosphatase levels is common.

X-ray studies. The chest X-ray appearance of miliary tuberculosis is often typical. Miliary shadowing is unusual in other diseases, but may occur in allergic alveolitis, sarcoidosis or histoplasmosis. X-ray studies reveal no abnormality in most cases of occult tuberculosis.

Sputum examination. There is rarely a significant production of sputum and, even if there is, it is unusual to see or culture mycobacteria from it. In the absence of sputum the overnight accumulation of gastric contents may be aspirated and sent for microscopy and culture.

The tuberculin test. Except in severely debilitated patients this is strongly positive. If negative, it should be repeated after 2 or 3 weeks. In occult tuberculosis it may be the only objective evidence of the nature of the disease. If the tuberculin test is negative more than once, alternative diagnoses such as drug fever, reticulosis or brucellosis should be considered.

Biopsies.   The liver biopsy reveals granulomata in patients with miliary tuberculosis and in about half of patients with occult disease. Biopsy of enlarged lymph nodes may also be helpful.

In a few cases mycobacteria can be cultured from biopsy material, or from bone-marrow aspirate, but not all cases of disseminated tuberculosis can be confirmed bacteriologically.

'Trial of therapy'.   This should only be carried out when all tests for the common kinds of tuberculosis, including examination of sputum, gastric aspirate and early morning urine, have been carried out on three occasions. (The tuberculin test will usually have been positive on the first occasion, and need not be repeated.) Full antituberculous therapy should be given. A definite response usually occurs within 7 days, but in some cases is delayed for 2 or 3 weeks. A trial of therapy should not be abandoned, therefore, in less than 1 month.

Reactivated (post-primary) tuberculosis

This is the form of tuberculosis which typically results in exuberant granuloma formation. The large granulomata caseate and break down, causing extensive tissue destruction and releasing many mycobacteria. Erosion of blood vessels by granuloma may cause bloodstream dissemination of organisms and result in miliary disease or in tuberculous meningitis.

Three quarters of cases of reactivated tuberculosis are pulmonary tuberculosis, but one-tenth of these cases will also have tuberculous disease in another body system, commonly a kidney, sometimes a bone or joint. (Fig. 20).

Clinical features of pulmonary tuberculosis
Post-primary pulmonary tuberculosis is the most commonly seen of all types.

The typical symptoms of tuberculosis are accompanied by cough and, often, by production of purulent sputum.

The cavitating lesion is usually in the upper lobe of one lung but, because it is patchy, it may not produce typical physical signs such as dullness on percussion, altered voice conduction or reduced breath sounds. Very extensive lesions can exist in the absence of physical signs. Bizarre signs, such as whispering pectoriloquy and aegophony, are extremely unusual. A few crepitations, or a small patch of dullness to percussion and reduced breath sounds, are the most that can be demonstrated in many cases.

Granuloma may erode blood vessels, resulting in haemoptysis, which is occasionally severe and life-threatening. Caseous material may discharge into the pleura, causing an empyema, or into the bronchial tree, to

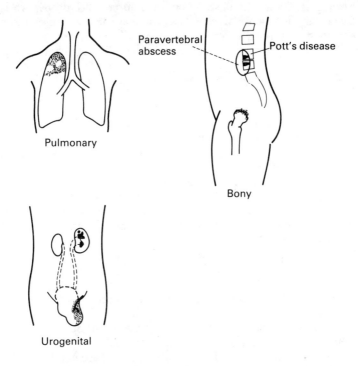

Fig. 20. Manifestations of postprimary tuberculosis.

cause tuberculous bronchopneumonia with widespread nodular shadow-ing on the chest X-ray.

Rupture of a cavity may lead to pneumothorax or bronchopleural fistula.

Occasionally secondary infection develops within the cavities. This produces an increase in volume and purulence of the sputum. Anaerobic infection causes an unpleasant, rancid fetor.

Urogenital tuberculosis
The caseating granuloma develops in a kidney, beginning in a single pyramid, deforming the calyx of the collecting system and discharging mycobacteria into the renal pelvis. Granulomata then develop in the ureter and later in the bladder. Spread may occur into the vas deferens, seminal vesicles and epididymis. Few patients present until infection of the lower urinary tract occurs. The commonest presentation is with frequency of micturition and dysuria. Haematuria may draw attention to the urinary tract early in the disease and occasionally renal colic results

from granulomatous obstruction of a ureter. Hydronephrosis can develop in the absence of renal colic, and may cause loin discomfort. Presentation with renal failure is rare.

Tuberculous epididymitis presents with unilateral induration, redness and swelling of the scrotum. Pain is not often severe. Cavitation may lead to formation of a 'cold abscess' and eventually to a discharging sinus.

Bone and joint disease

Almost any bone or joint can be affected. Commonly the end of a bone and its adjacent joint are both involved. In children the hip is most often affected but in all age-groups the hip, knee, wrist, elbow, shoulder and spine are all joints that can be attacked by tuberculosis. Pain and limitation of movement precede effusion and redness.

An effusion is common; in the wrist there may be effusion into the tendon sheaths. Purulent material can often be aspirated and contains a mixture of neutrophils and lymphocytes, as well as many organisms.

In spinal tuberculosis, the intervertebral disc is soon destroyed, and lesions then appear in the two adjacent vertebrae.

Female genital tuberculosis

Presumably due to bloodborne infection, disease begins in the fallopian tube and spreads to the endometrium. The cervix and vagina are rarely affected. In a minority of patients obstruction of the affected fallopian tube leads to the formation of a 'cold abscess'.

Symptoms are few and vague. Abdominal discomfort, mild, white vaginal discharge and infertility are the most common complaints. Menorrhagia may draw attention to the genital tract. Tubo-ovarian abscess presents with acute abdominal pain.

Gastrointestinal tuberculosis

This is a rare and difficult diagnosis. Any part of the alimentary tract can be affected by granulomatous, ulcerating lesions which are macroscopically like those of Crohn's disease. Presentation is often with abdominal pain and vague ill-health. Surgical and biopsy techniques are the usual means of diagnosis, though *M. tuberculosis* can be recovered from stool cultures in some cases.

Diagnosis of post-primary tuberculosis

Blood examination.   As usual in tuberculosis, this is often unhelpful, showing only a modest elevation of the ESR and disturbances of the liver function tests. In advanced pulmonary tuberculosis debility is common and the albumin level is then low. The serum sodium is also often low in these cases, though the reason for this is not clear.

X-ray examination.   Chest X-ray should be carried out in all patients because of the high frequency of pulmonary disease even when disease also exists in other sites. A typical fluffy, ill-defined, patchy shadow is seen in the apex of a lung. Cavities appear as round lucencies of various size. Bilateral involvement is not uncommon in advanced disease.

An element of healing can occur, visible as calcification, or as distortion of the mediastinum due to fibrosis. Small pleural effusions are common in severe cases.

In renal tuberculosis the intravenous urogram (IVP or IVU) is an indispensable diagnostic tool. The earliest sign is distension of one calyx, but renal cavitation and ureteric obstruction may be seen later. If one kidney cannot be seen, retrograde ureterography is necessary to demonstrate possible granulomatous ureteric stricture.

Abnormal radiographic features in bony tuberculosis develop some weeks after the initial symptoms. If the first X-rays are normal and symptoms persist, further films should be obtained after 3 or 4 weeks. The typical appearance is that of chronic osteomyelitis. Even the narrow disc space and destruction of adjacent vertebae in spinal tuberculosis is not pathognomonic, and further investigation is usually required to confirm the diagnosis (and to exclude staphylococcal infection or other causes of osteomyelitis).

Smears and cultures. Smears of sputum, gastric aspirate, sediment from centrifuged early morning urine or of caseous material from bone lesions will usually reveal mycobacteria if infection is present. A proportion of smears, particularly of urine, are negative but culture will confirm the presence of mycobacteria and allow identification and sensitivity testing. Culture of mycobacteria takes an average of 3 or 4 weeks (longer in partly treated cases) and sensitivity testing takes a further 4–6 weeks.

Examination of biopsies. Biopsy of bone lesions is usually required to confirm the diagnosis, but a positive smear or culture from a joint effusion may obviate this.

Endometrial curettage is necessary for the diagnosis of female genital tuberculosis. Granulomata are present in the premenstrual endometrium, but are discharged during menstruation. Culture of curettings (or sometimes of menstrual blood) will confirm the presence of mycobacteria.

The tuberculin test. This is strongly positive except in debilitated patients.

Treatment of tuberculosis

The principles of treatment are the same in all three types of tuberculosis. *Mycobacterium tuberculosis* is capable of developing resistance to a single drug in as short a time as 1 month, so at least two effective drugs must be given simultaneously to protect one another from the development of resistance. About 5% of *M. tuberculosis*, depending on the racial and social group involved, are resistant to one or more of the commonly used drugs. It is customary, therefore, to commence treatment with three drugs (triple therapy) so that at least two are effective, and to continue with two effective drugs when the sensitivities of the organism are known.

Drugs used in the treatment of tuberculosis

Rifampicin (first-line drug).   This is a powerful mycobacteriocidal drug which kills fast- and slow-growing mycobacteria both within and outside the cells. If it is used throughout the course of treatment, it reduces the previously necessary 18 month's therapy by several months.

Side-effects include reversible hepatocellular disturbance. A rise in transaminase levels to two or three times normal is usual when treatment is commenced. This usually improves after 3 or 4 weeks. Occasionally the abnormality continues to increase and dosage must be discontinued, or liver failure may follow. The appearance of bile in the urine is also an indication to discontinue dosage.

A small proportion of patients develop fever, myalgia and malaise ('flu-like syndrome) when taking rifampicin. This does not improve, and is an indication for discontinuation of dosage.

Renal failure occurs extremely rarely and usually after intermittent or erratic dosage, which makes all side-effects of rifampicin more likely and more severe.

Oral dose for adult over 60 kg, 600 mg daily as a morning dose; adult below 60 kg, 450 mg daily; child 10–20 mg/kg daily (maximum 600 mg). Metabolites make the urine appear brick-red in most patients.

Isoniazid (first-line drug).   A powerful drug which is well absorbed and reaches good tissue levels.

Side-effects include peripheral neuropathy (prevented by giving pyridoxine) and, rarely, hepatocellular liver damage.

Adult dose 300 mg daily in single or divided dose, orally. Child's dose 6 mg/kg daily (also available as injection).

Ethambutol (first-line drug).   Very effective drug whose only significant drawback is the dose-related ocular effect of central scotoma, affecting first colour vision and eventually visual acuity. Dose should be reduced in renal impairment and discontinued if visual defects occur.

Adult dose 15 mg/kg as a single daily dose orally (25 mg/kg if given as continuation therapy with only one other drug). Child's dose 35 mg/kg daily (not recommended below age 6).

Pyrazinamide (alternative or additional first-line drug).   A bactericidal drug which penetrates the meninges well.

Side-effects include hepatocellular damage, urticaria, sideroblastic anaemia and vomiting. *Not* effective against *M. bovis.*
Dose 20–30 mg/kg daily, orally (maximum 3 g).

Streptomycin (alternative first-line drug).   Unfortunately, this must be given by intramuscular injection. It is not hepatotoxic, so is useful in patients with liver disorder.

Major side-effects are rare with correct dose. Dosage *must* be reduced in renal impairment. Deafness and renal damage can occur, as with other aminoglycosides.

Dose for adult of 60 kg or more is 1.0 g daily as a single injection. Over age 40 or below 60 kg, 750 mg daily. Small patients may be given 500 mg daily.

Second-line drugs.   These are used for multiply-resistant organisms and for patients who cannot tolerate first-line drugs. Patients who have previously been incompletely treated are most likely to harbour resistant organisms. Available drugs are: ethionamide, prothionamide, aminosalicylic acid (PAS) and cycloserine. All have a high incidence of side-effects.

Dosage regimens
1. Rifampicin   } for 9 months in pulmonary tuberculosis. Probably
   Isoniazid   } 15–18 months in other types of disease.
   Ethambutol for first 2 months
   This is ideal and is the recommended regimen in Britain.
2. Isoniazid   }
   Ethambutol   } for 18 months (check colour vision 3-monthly)
   Streptomycin for first 3 months
   This is a good alternative if rifampicin cannot be used because of toxicity or expense.

Immunization
Active immunization is possible with live bacilli (Bacillus Calmette–Guérin or BCG). In some countries it is given to neonates; in Britain it is offered to tuberculin-negative children at age 10–13 years. It is little used in the United States of America.

Experience suggests that protection varies in different areas of the world. In Europe, significant protection lasts for about 15 years. In North India the protective effect is uncertain.

The vaccine *must* be given intradermally (intracutaneously). Subcutaneous injection will cause a persistent abscess, which requires needle aspiration if it does not heal spontaneously.

There is some evidence that BCG can protect to a variable degree against *Mycobacterium leprae* in endemic areas.

14

Some Zoonoses: Toxoplasmosis, Brucellosis, Anthrax and Plague

Introduction
A zoonosis is a disease of animals whose natural cycle has been interrupted by man. Prolonged close contact with animals is usually necessary for the transmission of the disease and many zoonoses therefore occur in those with occupations involving animals, their carcases, hides, excreta or other products. Domestic contact with animals is a less frequent means of contracting a zoonosis. Some animal diseases have an uneven distribution in different countries, so that travellers are sometimes at risk of contracting a disease which is rare in their own country.

Some zoonoses have already been mentioned in previous chapters; orf, cat-scratch disease and cowpox (see Chapter 2), Q fever (see Chapter 4), leptospirosis and rabies (see Chapters 8 and 9). These have been discussed in the context of their differential diagnoses. The examples of zoonosis discussed in this chapter have earned special mention because they are sufficiently common or, in some cases severe, to present the occasional diagnostic challenge to the general physician.

Toxoplasmosis

Epidemiology
Toxoplasmosis is an infection due to the protozoan parasite *Toxoplasma gondii*. This organism is widespread in warm-blooded creatures, in whose tissues it survives as intracellular 'cysts'. Carnivores probably acquire infection by eating infected prey. Members of the cat family are known to excrete infectious oocysts of *Toxoplasma* in their faeces for some time after infection, and the oocysts can survive for many weeks in damp conditions, though they are killed by desiccation.

Two routes of infection have been proposed for man. In countries where raw or lightly cooked meat is often eaten infection may be acquired in the diet, while in other countries contact with the faeces of domestic cats may result in accidental ingestion of cysts. Unfortunately, few patients can remember contact with either source of infection. Differences in dietary habit may, for example, explain the relatively low incidence of toxoplasmosis in the United Kingdom compared with the rest of Europe. Even in the United Kingdom, however, nearly half of the adult urban population have serological evidence of past infection.

Clinical features
Many infections must be trivial or asymptomatic, as few people with serological evidence of infection can remember having an illness. Of acute symptomatic infections about three-quarters present as a glandular fever syndrome. There is moderate fever, marked malaise and lassitude, and enlargement of a group of lymph nodes or a single node. Widespread lymphadenopathy is unusual, as the cervical nodes are often affected and the inguinal nodes rarely. Few patients have a palpable spleen.

Uncommon acute presentations include fever of unknown origin, local disease in skin, breast or other tissue, hepatitis, myocarditis, meningitis and encephalitis.

In well-established infection or late after infection uveitis is common. Although symptomatic iridocyclitis can occur, the more usual picture is one of insidiously advancing chorioretinitis which only becomes evident when there is a large visual field defect or when macular involvement causes blurred vision. On fundoscopy white areas of sclera can be seen where the choroid has been destroyed, and a black, ragged edge of choroid outlines the lesion. In the very early stages, only pale areas of oedema are visible in the fundus.

Unusually severe and persistent toxoplasmosis sometimes results from congenital infection (see Chapter 16) and from infection in patients with defective cell-mediated immunity. Glandular toxoplasmosis can confuse the clinical picture in Hodgkin's disease or leukaemia.

Diagnosis
The white blood cell count shows a mild atypical mononucleosis in many patients with acute toxoplasmosis, but the Paul-Bunnell test is negative.

Serology.   The traditional diagnostic test is Sabin's toxoplasma dye test in which antibodies in the patient's blood inhibit the uptake of vital stain by live organisms. Many laboratories now use haemagglutination, immunofluorescent, or complement fixation tests which do not require live organisms.

Patients with acute infection often have dye test titres of 1:1000 or more, or rising titres in paired sera. Those with uveitis tend to have titres in a lower range. IgM antibodies can be detected for 6–12 months after infection.

Treatment
It is rarely necessary to treat toxoplasmosis other than symptomatically as the illness usually resolves gradually over a period of weeks. Specific

therapy may, however, be indicated in cases with central nervous system disease, cardiac involvement or immune deficiency states. There is no entirely satisfactory therapy, but high-dose co-trimoxazole or pyrimethamine–sulphonamide combinations have both been used with a measure of success. This treatment probably does not eradicate all intracellular *Toxoplasma* cysts, so prolonged dosage, and maintenace therapy may be required to avoid relapse.

Severe uveitis is often treated with topical corticosteroid drops which reduce the inflammatory response without apparently worsening the course of the disease. Expert ophthalmological supervision is recommended, however.

Brucellosis

Epidemiology

Brucellosis is a disease of animals which is often associated with genital disease and abortion of the fetus. The responsible organisms are Gram-negative coccobacilli of the genus *Brucella*. *B. abortus* causes contagious abortion in cows, *B. melitensis* affects goats, *B. suis* affects pigs. Other organisms, such as *B. ovis* and *B. canis*, affecting sheep and dogs, are hardly ever seen in human cases.

Infection can be acquired by close contact with placentas, genital secretions, products of conception, carcases or blood. The disease is most often seen therefore in farmers, herdsmen, meat handlers and veterinary surgeons whose occupation involves them in such contact. Organisms are also excreted in milk, so that users of unpasteurized milk or cream may be at risk. Tourists may consume such milk inadvertently in farm guesthouses or hotels. Mature yogurt and cheese are usually too acidic for the organism to survive, and rarely transmit infection.

In the United Kingdom, a scheme to eradicate *B. abortus* from cattle herds has led to a parallel fall in human brucellosis and most of the cases which occur have been contracted abroad (Fig. 21).

Clinical features

There is an enormous range of symptomatology associated with brucellosis but there are three main types of disease.

Acute brucellosis.   This can be an extremely severe and disabling disease. If due to *B. melitensis* it is often known as Malta fever.

The incubation period generally falls within the range of 1–4 weeks but may be much longer. There is then an abrupt onset of high swinging fever, profuse sweating, chills or rigors and often headache, myalgia and arthralgia. Malaise and exhaustion are severe even though the patient may not seem seriously ill on examination. Physical examination rarely reveals any abnormality though one patient in ten may have a palpable spleen.

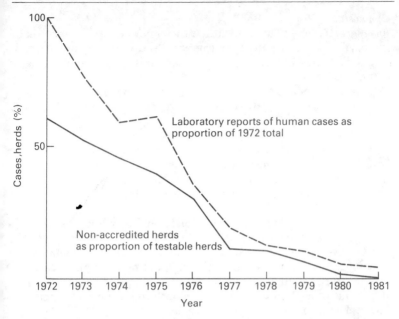

Fig. 21. Decline of human brucellosis in England and Wales with control in cattle herds (CDSC).

The acute illness tends to subside spontaneously in 1–3 months but relapse or progression to chronic disease is common.

Chronic brucellosis. The variable symptomatology of this form of brucellosis presents a difficult diagnostic problem. It may follow an acute illness or develop insidiously without prior warning. A low-grade fever is associated with extreme fatigue, malaise and lassitude. Profuse sweating, particularly at night, is common. Associated features include myalgia, arthralgia, arthritis of large or small joints, abdominal pain, uveitis, orchitis and weight loss. Endocarditis occasionally develops. Not surprisingly, depression is frequently seen and can further confuse the diagnosis.

In some cases the fever waxes and wanes over a period of weeks with days or weeks of improvement between exacerbations. This form of brucellosis is known as undulant fever.

Reactive illness. This form of illness, not truly an infection, is a form of hypersensitivity to *Brucella* antigens which develops after frequent exposure or past infection. It begins soon after exposure to antigenic material and comprises a disabling combination of fever, sweating and malaise, sometimes with a rash. It subsides on removal of the stimulus.

Diagnosis
Blood examination.   In acute disease there may be a modest neutrophil leukocytosis, though in the chronic form a neutropenia is more common. The ESR is modestly raised in many cases but is not always abnormal in chronic cases.

Blood cultures can provide the diagnosis in either form of disease but must be incubated for 6–10 weeks as the organism, particularly *B. abortus* is very slow-growing.

Other measures.   Chronic brucellosis causes granuloma formation in lymph nodes, liver, kidney and other organs. Lymph node or liver biopsy may show such granulomata on histology and may produce positive cultures. Culture of bone marrow is also worthwhile.

Serology.   This may be the only available means of diagnosis but difficulties of interpretation are often encountered. Four types of antibodies can be investigated by direct agglutination test, indirect agglutination (Coomb's) test, complement fixation test and radioimmunoassay.

The direct agglutination titre is often raised to 1:320 or more early in the course of acute disease, and the other titres are usually somewhat lower. The titres fall as the illness improves.

In chronic disease all of the titres may be modestly raised to 1:40 or 1:80 but insignificant titres have been reported even in cases with positive blood cultures. Such titres must therefore be interpreted in the light of the clinical and epidemiological situation.

False-positive titres are also seen in patients with hypersensitivity to *Brucella* antigens but without infection. This can cause great difficulty in those with regular occupational exposure to antigen.

Caution.   Because of the uncertain clinical picture and serodiagnostic features of brucellosis, other causes of chronic debility should always merit consideration in suspected cases. The differential diagnosis includes tuberculosis, toxoplasmosis, cytomegalic inclusion disease, occult malignancy and psychiatric disorders.

Treatment
Acute brucellosis.   The treatment of choice is tetracycline. It is given in high dosage for 4 weeks. In order to avoid relapse or chronicity it is advisable to repeat the course after a break of 2 weeks. Many physicians also recommend that streptomycin be added to the first 2 or 3 weeks' therapy during the first course of tetracycline.

Chronic brucellosis.   This is usually treated with a long course of tetracycline. A minimum of 8 weeks' therapy is usually given and courses of 6 months or more may be required in long-standing cases.

If tetracycline cannot be tolerated or has failed on two occasions co-trimoxazole is a good alternative.

Prevention
Effective vaccines are available for use in animals but are not yet available for human use.

Pasteurization of milk and cream is effective in destroying *Brucella spp.* Unpasteurized milk is consumed by farmers and herdsmen worldwide and is available as a 'health food' in some western countries. In the United Kingdom it is available commercially as 'green top' milk. Eradication of brucellosis from herds, however, has greatly reduced the risk of infection by untreated milk.

Anthrax

Epidemiology
Anthrax is a disease mainly of ungulates: cattle, sheep, horses, goats and pigs. It is due to infection with *Bacillus anthracis*, an aerobic, Gram-positive, spore-bearing bacillus with a worldwide distribution. Spores may persist in pasture for many years after occupation by infected animals, and ingestion of spores while grazing is a well-known cause of infection in animals. It is also possible that insects can spread infection by biting.

Human infection is most likely in those who have close contact with sick animals, hides, bones and carcases. Such exposure occurs in wool-sorters, in the animal hair and hide industries and in the bonemeal and glue industries. Hair shaving brushes have been known to cause non-occupational infection.

The disease is usually acquired by inoculation of spores into a lesion on exposed skin but 2 or 3% of cases follow inhalation or ingestion of spores.

Clinical features
Cutaneous anthrax (malignant pustule). A painless red swelling appears usually on the hand, head or neck. Over a week or so it develops a rim of vesicles which become haemorrhagic and eventually crust to form a dark scab, the black eschar. Extensive, non-tender, non-pitting oedema is usually a striking feature, and the local lymph nodes are often enlarged. Constitutional symptoms are few and over half of cases tend to heal spontaneously, the scab disappearing within 1 or 2 weeks, though the oedema usually persists for much longer.

If untreated, the remainder of cases will progress to septicaemic disease with high fever and prostration. Small blood vessels are occluded by masses of organisms, causing damage to the brain and other organs and leading to extensive thrombosis. Septicaemic disease is usually fatal.

Pulmonary anthrax (woolsorter's disease).   Following inhalation of large numbers of spores, a widespread pneumonia occurs with consolidation, haemoptysis, and mediastinitis due to spread of infection from enlarged mediastinal lymph nodes. Eventually septicaemia and death ensue.

Gastrointestinal anthrax.   This is extremely rare and follows ingestion of large numbers of spores. It presents with severe watery, blood-stained diarrhoea.

Diagnosis

Blood examination.   There is little abnormality of the blood count in simple cutaneous anthrax but severe disease is accompanied by a neutrophil leukocytosis.

Microbiology.   Smears of vesicle fluid or exudate show numerous organisms in cutaneous anthrax. In pulmonary or gastrointestinal disease smears of sputum or faeces produce a similar result.

Culture of these specimens, or of blood, will usually confirm the diagnosis.

Treatment

B. anthracis is sensitive to many antibiotics. The treatment of choice is parenteral benzylpenicillin, but erythromycin, tetracycline, streptomycin or chloramphenicol may also be used. Mortality is extremely low in treated cases and usually results from major thrombosis complicating septicaemia.

Prevention

Animal hair can be treated chemically, and bones or bonemeal can be autoclaved to reduce the risk to handlers. Hides, however, cannot be easily treated and many are imported from endemic areas.

Workers at risk of anthrax can be immunized with a killed vaccine. Port workers and workers in the hide and leather industry are encouraged to be immunized and are usually offered regular immunization under their various occupational health schemes.

Effective vaccines are available for animal use. Cases of animal anthrax are reported to the State Veterinary Services in many countries, and special arrangements are made for safe disposal of carcases.

Plague

Epidemiology

This is a disease of rodents, particularly of rats. It is caused by the Gram-negative rod *Yersinia pestis*, which is transferred from rat to rat by fleas. Rat fleas may bite humans who come into close contact with the rats, and the bite of an infected flea is the cause of human disease. Sporadic cases and small outbreaks of plague are occasionally reported from the Far East, Africa, South America and the United States of America. They occur in both rural and urban evironments when humans are in close contact with rats, or rarely, other rodents.

Clinical features and diagnosis
Human disease is usually septicaemia. It is known as bubonic plague because of the large lymph node swellings which accompany it. The incubation period varies, but is usually 2–4 days. High fever, prostration and pain in the affected lymph nodes occur suddenly. The buboes often discharge plus.

In rare cases there is also severe pneumonia, and patients with this can spread disease by the airborne route.

Diagnosis is made on clinical grounds, and confirmed by identification of *Y. pestis* in lymph node aspirate, blood or, in pneumonic cases, sputum.

Treatment
This should be prompt, as the mortality is then very low. Intravenous streptomycin is usually given, chloramphenicol and tetracycline are also effective.

Prevention
Control of rodents is most important, but inactivated vaccines are available for laboratory workers and others at high risk of exposure.

Drugs mentioned in this chapter

Drug	Indication	Usage and precautions
Benzylpenicillin	Anthrax	Cutaneous disease: adult dose 600 mg to 1.2 g (1.0–2.0 mega units) 6-hourly by intra-muscular or intravenous injection; child's dose is a quarter to half of adult dose; in dis-seminated disease, 16–20 mega units daily may be given
Chloramphenicol	Plague	Adult dose initially 2.0 g 6-hourly orally or intravenously, followed by 1.0 g 8-hourly for 7 days after fever resolves; child's dose 100 mg/kg daily, then 50 mg/kg daily, both in divided doses

Co-trimoxazole	Alternative drug for use in brucellosis	Adult dose 960–1440 mg (2 to 3 tablets) 12-hourly orally; maintenance dose 960 mg once or twice daily for 6–12 weeks; child's dose 6 weeks to 5 months 120 mg twice daily; 6 months to 5 years 240 mg twice daily; 6–12 years 480 mg twice daily
Streptomycin	Acute brucellosis, used with tetracycline	Adult dose 1.0 g daily in one or two divided doses intramuscularly for the first 2 weeks of therapy; patients under 60 kg 0.75 g daily
	Plague (drug of choice)	Adult dose 1.0 g 6-hourly for 48 hours, then 1.0–1.5 g daily for 7 days, intramuscular injections
Tetracycline	Acute brucellosis	Adult dose 500 mg 6-hourly orally for two courses each of 4 weeks, separated by 2 weeks without treatment
	Chronic brucellosis	Adult dose 500 mg 6-hourly orally for 2–4 weeks, then 250 mg 6-hourly; in children tetracycline can stain developing teeth, but it may be given in a quarter to half of the adult dose if unavoidable

15

'Childhood' Infectious Diseases

Introduction
Not very many years ago childhood diseases, including scarlet fever, whooping cough and gastroenteritis, would have filled a major part of this book. Many recent developments have modified this now old-fashioned view of infectious diseases. Better living standards have reduced the seriousness of measles. The severity of scarlet fever seems to have decreased, and preventive medicine including immunization has modified the incidence of several diseases. Most must now take their place within the differential diagnosis of similar diseases in all age groups. Those diseases discussed here are those associated with rashes or other eruptions and are commonly known as 'childhood exanthematous diseases'.

These exanthematous diseases are systemic viral infections all of which have a distinct respiratory component, and which are transmitted mainly by droplet infection. In the absence of preventive measures they are quite highly infectious and easily spread among nursery and school children who have lost their maternally derived antibodies. In the general population 80–90% of adults have serological evidence of past infection. Children born to women who lack antibodies can suffer infection in the neonatal period or in early infancy. In normal circumstances infection is acquired from a patient in the infectious stages of the disease and asymptomatic carriers are not thought to exist.

Not all of these diseases are endemic worldwide. Chickenpox is not often encountered in the Philippines and other Pacific regions, while rubella is relatively uncommon in Asia. People who come from these areas to live in western or Australasian countries are often susceptible to the exanthematous diseases and unfortunately can suffer quite severe attacks, as adults are more susceptible to severe or complicated illness than children.

Measles

Epidemiology
This is a viral respiratory infection due to a morbillivirus, related to parainfluenza viruses. It is highly infectious and is transmitted by infected droplets which enter the conjunctival or respiratory mucosa. Children are susceptible by the age of 6–12 months, when they have lost

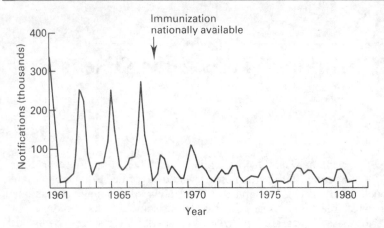

Fig. 22. Effect of immunization on measles epidemics in England and Wales (CDSC).

maternal antibodies, and can contract the infection from school contacts or from older sibs. The long-recognized 2-yearly epidemics of measles have now been suppressed by immunization (Fig. 22).

Clinical features
Incubation period.   This is usually about 11 days with a range of 10–14 days.

Prodromal illness.   This is a distinct feature of the disease, lasting for 3 or 4 days. It takes the form of a catarrhal illness with high fever, reddened conjunctivae, sore mouth and nasal discharge. Patients are often miserable and irritable, possibly because of mild encephalitis, and febrile convulsions are common. There is usually a repetitive cough which may be croupy. Mild diarrhoea is not unusual and probably reflects 'catarrhal' inflammation of the gastrointestinal mucosa.

An internal rash or *enanthem*, consisting of Koplik's spots, is seen in the mouth: irregular lesions like small breadcrumbs or salt crystals on a red background appear on the buccal mucosa, usually opposite the lower molars.

Exanthematous phase.   The rash begins behind the ears and in the hairline, and spreads down the face and body, reaching the feet in 2 or 3 days. It is exaggerated in the napkin and other warm areas. The lesions are large and maculopapular, being particularly 'blotchy' on the face. In severe cases and in some Asian races there may be a marked petechial element. The Koplik's spots disappear during the first few days of the rash.

The cough continues as the rash develops and many crepitations may be heard on auscultation of the lungs. These findings indicate the presence of a giant-cell interstitial pneumonitis which will resolve when the rash passes its peak.

On the third or fourth day the bright pink rash begins to change its colour to orange-brown. This change, known as staining, is characteristic though it sometimes occurs in other severe rashes. The brown staining gradually fades during the next week or so.

Other features. Lymphadenopathy is quite common, especially in children. It can occur during the prodrome and the eruption of the rash. Involvement of abdominal lymph nodes occasionally produces the picture of mesenteric lymphadenitis and causes diagnostic confusion until the rash appears.

Encephalitis is probably common but mild during the prodromal period. Post-infectious encephalitis develops as the rash reaches its peak, and usually presents as drowsiness and irritability. Although it is rare, affecting only about 0.1% of cases, it can be very severe, and intellectual or neurological sequelae persist in a high proportion of cases.

Haemorrhagic measles is a rare severe infection with petechiae, ecchymoses and sometimes platelet consumption due to severe vasculitis. Evidence of renal and hepatic disturbance is often found in these cases.

The infectious period
This is from 2 days before prodromal illness to the appearance of staining of the rash.

Complications
Secondary bacterial infection. Bacterial chest infection is the most common complication of measles and can be a cause of death in debilitated children. The persistence of cough and appearance of purulent sputum when the rash is staining are the typical signs. As in influenza, *Staphylococcus aureus* is a frequent invader of the lungs, which are already damaged by viral infection.

Acute otitis media is a consequence of the catarrhal stage of the disease when the Eustachian tube easily becomes blocked.

Subacute sclerosing panencephalitis (SSPE). This is a very rare complication which occurs in children who have had measles before the age of 2 (see Chapter 9).

Diagnosis
This is usually obvious from the clinical features, though prolonged prodromata or atypical features do occur in some sporadic cases.

A rising titre of complement-fixing antibodies in paired sera is strong evidence of recent infection.

The chest X-ray is normal unless secondary bacterial infection has occurred, when pneumonic changes may be seen.

Electroencephalography shows non-specific changes during the prodrome and in post-infectious encephalitis. Specific changes are seen in SSPE.

Treatment
Most patients require only supportive treatment. Early bacterial secondary infections may be treated with oral antibiotics such as erythromycin, amoxycillin, ampicillin or co-trimoxazole. The likely presence of staphylococci should be borne in mind, and cloxacillin, flucloxacillin or a cephalosporin used if indicated.

Prophylaxis
Active immunization with live attenuated vaccine is offered to British children during the second year of life. In the United States of America it is required before school entry as part of a measles eradication programme.

Passive immunization with human normal immunoglobulin can be offered to susceptible patients endangered by exposure to measles. Treatment should be given within 3 days after exposure.

Rubella

Epidemiology
This is a viral infection caused by a rubivirus, a member of the Togaviridae. It is almost always brief and mild, and hardly ever causes long-term sequelae in healthy children or adults. Mild or subclinical infection is common, so that clinical features are unlikely to be a reliable basis for studying the epidemiology of the disease. Serological surveys show that in the absence of immunization up to 15% of western populations remained susceptible to rubella during early adult life.

The importance of rubella lies in its ability to cause transplacental infection of the fetus, resulting in severe developmental abnormalities.

It is spread by droplet transmission.

Clinical features
Incubation period.   This is usually 17 or 18 days, but may be from 2 to 3 weeks.

Prodromal illness.   This is not usually seen except in some adults who suffer fever and malaise for a day or two before the rash appears.

Exanthematous phase.   This may present as any or all of several respiratory features including a gritty-feeling soreness and pinkness of the conjunctivae, mild-to-moderate sore throat, moderate enlargement of cervical and occipital lymph nodes, and rash. The rash accompanies the other features or follows within 24 hours, beginning on the forehead or face, and quickly spreading to the rest of the body. It is composed of small maculopapular elements which sometimes coalesce to produce an erythema very similar to the punctate erythema of scarlet fever (or of toxic shock syndrome), from which it must be differentiated. An enanthem of petechial lesions on the palate, called Forcheimer spots, is sometimes seen.

The whole illness seldom lasts more than 3 or 4 days, but may be longer with high fever, headache and malaise in adults.

The infectious period. This is from 1 week before the rash to about 1 week after, though virus has been isolated from pharyngeal secretions for up to 2 weeks after the appearance of the rash.

Complications

Arthralgia and arthritis. Pain in the finger and wrist joints occurs in a significant number of young women and sometimes in other patients. It usually begins when the rash and other symptoms are subsiding, and may last for a week or more. In rare cases large-joint arthritis with effusion is seen, but like arthralgia it is self-limiting and without long-term sequelae.

Encephalitis. This is rare, as is meningoencephalitis. It may begin during or after the rash and, although it can be severe, it rarely causes any long-term deficit.

Fetal infection. Fetal infection and damage can occur at any stage of pregnancy, but is particularly severe in the first trimester. If rubella is suspected in a pregnant woman, energetic efforts should be made to confirm the diagnosis without delay so that arrangements can be made for termination of pregnancy if indicated.

Diagnosis

This is usually based on a rising titre of antibodies in paired sera. Complement-fixing antibodies are less reliable than haemagglutination-inhibiting antibodies (HAI), which are most frequently estimated in Britain. For prompt diagnosis of active or recent infection IgM antibodies can be sought.

Treatment

Only symptomatic treatment is available. Soluble aspirin and other non-steroidal anti-inflammation agents (NSAID) are useful in controlling arthralgia.

Prophylaxis
The value of immunoglobulin in preventing the development of rubella after exposure is now in doubt, as large doses given however promptly have failed to protect. Immunoglobulin prophylaxis is therefore not often recommended, though it may be offered to a susceptible woman who wishes to complete her pregnancy after exposure to rubella.

Active immunization.   This is with a live attenuated vaccine and is offered to all schoolgirls between the ages of 10 and 14 years. It may also be given to susceptible women of child-bearing age, who should be warned to avoid pregnancy for 3 months after immunization.

Chickenpox (varicella)

Epidemiology
This is the disease of primary infection with varicella-zoster virus, which is a member of the group of herpes viruses. Primary infection (chickenpox) is followed by a long period of latency during which the virus survives in the dorsal nerve ganglia. Fever, trauma or immune deficiency are thought to result in reactivation of the virus when circulating antibodies have diminished below a critical level, and herpes zoster then results.

Chickenpox is extremely infectious. It spreads by droplet transmission either in pharyngeal secretions or in vesicle fluid from cases of chickenpox or herpes zoster.

Clinical features
Incubation period.   This is usually 14–17 days, but may be from 11 to 25 days.

Prodromal illness.   This is rarely seen in children, but in adults it may take the form of 2 or 3 days' quite severe malaise and fever.

Exanthematous phase.   The rash appears first on the body and later on the face and proximal limbs. The distal limbs are relatively spared, so that the rash has a centripetal distribution. Although the lesions begin as papules they are usually first noticed at the vesicular stage, when they look like oval water drops with their long axis following the skin creases. Occasionally the first 'crop' of papules is noticed before any vesicles are present, causing diagnostic difficulty, but the papular stage seldom lasts more than a few hours. A generalized erythema may precede, or coexist with, the rash. In the next 3–6 days the vesicles progress to pustules and finally to dry scabs or crusts, while new crops of papules appear at intervals between the vesicles. As the rash gets older, the papular lesions become smaller and eventually fail to progress to the other stages. All of the remaining vesicles form crusts, which usually fall away without scarring.

Vesicles in the mouth and vulva may ulcerate and cause considerable discomfort.

Other features

Pneumonia.   This is a feature usually seen in adults, and it develops in parallel with the rash, which is often severe. Symptoms vary from moderate shortness of breath to severe respiratory difficulty with cough and haemoptysis. There is widespread focal alveolitis and auscultation may reveal coarse crepitations throughout the lung fields in severe cases.

The chest X-ray may be normal in mild cases, but usually shows widespread nodular opacities of varying size. These opacities persist and eventually calcify to produce the picture of 'chickenpox lung'.

Haemorrhagic chickenpox.   This severe disease is again more common in adults. Bleeding into the vesicles may be associated with the appearance of petechiae and ecchymoses elsewhere. Vasculitis can lead to necrosis of skin, especially of the fingers. Mucosal lesions in the mouth or gut may bleed profusely. In rare severe cases disseminated intravascular coagulation has been reported.

Encephalitis.   This is not uncommon, and is usually a benign focal encephalitis beginning as the rash resolves. It presents as vertigo and ataxia, with nystagmus and an abnormal Romberg's test, only rarely progressing to coma with cortical or pyramidal deficit. Even in the rare, severe cases, complete resolution often occurs in a matter of days.

The infectious period

This is from 3 or 4 days before the rash (usually about 10 days after exposure) to the time when all lesions are dry and crusted.

Complications

Secondary bacterial infection.   Skin infection can easily be introduced into scratched-off chickenpox lesions. *Staphylococcus aureus* is a common invader, resulting in impetigo and occasionally in bacteraemia. *Streptococcus pyogenes* and *Corynebacterium diphtheriae* are uncommon but well-recognized secondary invaders which can cause severe complications. Secondarily infected lesions may leave scars after healing.

Bacteraemia should be suspected if high fever persists for more than 3 or 4 days after the rash begins.

Caution.   Chickenpox is a dangerous infection in patients with defective cell-mediated immunity. Patients on immunosuppressive therapy, or with lymphocytic leukaemia or Hodgkin's disease, can develop a progressive severe disease with confluent rash, pneumonitis, encephalitis and renal impairment. Herpes zoster can also progress to generalized infection in these patients.

Diagnosis
This is usually evident on clinical and epidemiological grounds. Papular urticaria with a vesicular element may appear similar, but is often confined to the arms and legs. In some parts of the world rickettsialpox is a cause of vesicular skin lesions, but these are usually accompanied by distinct maculopapular lesions in the same patient.

Smallpox as a natural infection has now been eradicated but is still suspected from time to time. The lesions of smallpox are rounder and deeper than those of chickenpox and are more marked on the face and peripheries. Only one crop of lesions occurs. Specially designated laboratories are equipped to carry out electron microscopy, gel diffusion and virus culture in cases of doubt. (Procedure is as for viral haemorrhagic fevers; see Chapter 17.)

Rising titres of complement-fixing antibodies to varicella zoster virus can be detected in paired sera in both chickenpox and herpes zoster.

Treatment
The illness usually resolves in 1 or 2 weeks without specific treatment. In cases of haemorrhagic disease, pneumonitis or generalized progressive disease, the new antiviral drugs vidarabine or acyclovir can be given, and will often modify the course of the illness; indeed some impressive responses have been reported.

Impetiginized skin lesions can be treated with oral cloxacillin or flucloxacillin. Other bacterial infections and bacteraemias require vigorous parenteral treatment with appropriate antibiotics.

Prophylaxis
The development of chickenpox in susceptible individuals can often be prevented by zoster immune globulin (ZIG) given within 2 days of exposure.

Mumps

Epidemiology
This is a systemic viral infection in which virus is excreted in the saliva and the urine. Infection is by direct contact with saliva or by droplet transmission. Although mumps appears to be less infectious than some other childhood diseases, this may be because of the frequency of atypical and subclinical cases, for about 80% of adults in western countries have mumps antibodies whether or not they remember having typical mumps.

Clinical features
Incubation period.   This is usually 18–21 days, but varies from 2 to 4 weeks.

Salivary adenitis.   Inflammation of the parotid glands is the commonest and best-recognized feature of mumps, though inflammation of several other organs and systems also occurs, producing a variable spectrum of symptoms which may appear in any order.

Not all patients have salivary adenitis, but 80–90% do, and at least two-thirds of these have bilateral parotitis. The glands suddenly become grossly swollen and are usually tender. Stabbing pain on salivation is quite common and the opening of Stensen's duct is usually red and surrounded by oedema. The swelling of the two glands can occur a day or two apart or, in a minority of patients, only one gland is affected. Occasional patients have swelling of the mandibular glands, with or without parotitis. In most cases there is marked oedema of the facial tissues, especially under the chin. The oedema is lax, and vibrates if sharply tapped, like a soft jelly; it does not pit.

Meningitis and encephalitis.   These are not at all uncommon and may precede or follow the parotitis; occasionally they occur without other features of mumps. Mild encephalitis, appearing as extreme irritability, is probably quite common and a high proportion of sufferers have subtle neurological signs such as transiently extensor plantar responses. Meningitis is often severe, with pronounced meningism. It may present alone, but commonly appears when the initial parotitis has improved somewhat and the fever often appears to resolve before rising again as the headache begins. Illness rarely lasts for more than 4–7 days.

In very rare instances neurological sequelae follow encephalitis or meningitis. The most frequent of these is nerve deafness.

Orchitis.   Like meningitis this often occurs after initial improvement in the original illness, but can exist alone. It is usually seen in adult men, but occasionally occurs in prepubertal cases. The testicle swells to several times its usual size and is extremely painful. The epididymis is also swollen. About three-quarters of cases have unilateral disease and resolution rarely takes longer than a week; marked improvement occurs in 3 or 4 days. A few cases have prolonged inflammation for 6 weeks or more and these patients may suffer gradual slight atrophy of the testicle. Infertility only occurs in rare cases of severe bilateral atrophy.

Pancreatitis.   Mild abdominal tenderness with anorexia or vomiting is not uncommon, but severe acute pancreatitis with paralytic ileus is rare. Transient or permanent diabetes mellitus can follow such illness, and malabsorption with steatorrhoea has been reported. Rare cases of pancreatic pseudocyst are also seen.

Other features.   These include oophoritis, thyroiditis, hepatitis and myocarditis. Transient large joint arthritis may occur in young men. Thrombocytopenia is occasionally seen.

Diagnosis
Although the diagnosis is often suggested by epidemiological and clinical features, sporadic and atypical cases without parotitis can present problems.

In contrast to many viral infections, the white cell count in mumps is raised as often as it is normal, and when meningitis or orchitis occur there may be a neutrophil leukocytosis.

Parotitis.   This must be distinguished from bacterial or obstructive disease of the parotid and from sarcoidosis or idiopathic swellings (Mikulicz's syndrome). Although the serum amylase is raised in mumps, it is sometimes raised in other types of parotitis and pancreatitis.

Parotitis must also be distinguished from suppurative cervical lymphadenitis, especially in children. The fact that the swollen parotid gland envelops the angle of the mandible while a lymph node is usually deep to it, is helpful as is the presence of jelly-like oedema in mumps.

Meningitis.   This can also present with misleading features including neutrophil leukocytosis and a tendency for the cerebrospinal fluid sugar level to be unusually low. The cells in the CSF, however, are predominantly lymphocytes as would be expected.

Orchitis.   If this occurs in isolation it must be distinguished from torsion of the testicle; the axis of the swollen testicle is usually normal in mumps and displaced in torsion. Bacterial epididymitis and other viral orchitis, such as coxsackie infection, should also be considered.

Microbiological diagnosis.   This is commonly made by estimation of the 'S and V' antibody levels. These are complement-fixing antibodies. The soluble (S) antibody level reaches a peak within 2 weeks and is often raised when the patient presents. The viral (V) antibody rises more slowly and a significantly rising titre of V antibodies in paired sera, with a persistently high S antibody, indicates a recent infection.

Mumps virus is detectable in standard tissue cultures.

Treatment
No specific treatment is available. Adequate hydration and analgesia contribute greatly to the treatment of the acute or complicated illness.

Patients with pancreatitis may require intensive care with monitoring of fluid, electrolyte, calcium and glucose levels.

Prophylaxis
A live attenuated vaccine is available for immunization against mumps. It may be given to any individual over 1 year old, but it is not currently recommended for inclusion in British immunization programmes.

Some practitioners prescribe prednisolone for adult men with mumps in an attempt to prevent the occurrence of orchitis. There is little evidence, however, that this is effective.

Other Exanthematous Diseases

Many infectious diseases can present with rashes similar to those described above. Echovirus, coxsackie virus and E–B virus are all well-known examples. Bacteria such as pyogenic streptococci and staphylococci can produce toxic rashes similar to that of rubella, while influenza, Q fever, mycoplasma infections and syphilis are occasional causes of puzzling rashes.

Allergic rashes, particularly antibiotic-induced, can cause a confusing diagnostic picture when they appear in the course of another disease.

Two other diseases of small children are worthy of mention as they have a characteristic presentation with a rash. Both illnesses mainly affect preschool children up to the age of 2 or 3 years.

Roseola infantum or exanthem subitum

This disease is presumed to be a viral infection. It usually occurs sporadically, though outbreaks have been recorded in which the incubation period is 10 days or a little longer.

Illness begins with the abrupt onset of high fever. There are few physical signs except perhaps a reddened throat or mild catarrh, though irritability or a convulsion may result from the fever. After 3 or 4 days the fever suddenly drops and a rubelliform rash appears on the body, quickly spreading to the limbs and face. At this stage neutropenia is common. The rash usually disappears in 2 or 3 days. Mild cases may be very short-lived and atypical.

Slapped-cheek syndrome

This is very similar to roseola infantum. It begins with 2 or 3 days' fever and listlessness and ends with a rash. The rash is a blotchy erythema of the cheeks, which may even have a linear pattern like the mark of a hand after a slap.

Both illnesses are brief and require no special treatment.

Drugs mentioned in this chapter

The drugs used to treat secondary infections of the skin and of the respiratory tract are discussed in Chapters 2 to 4 (skin and mucous membrane infections, mouth and throat infections and respiratory infections).

Life-threatening chickenpox and its severe manifestations may be treated with antiviral agents. On the present evidence, acyclovir is probably the drug of choice.

Drug	Indication	Usage and precautions
Acyclovir	Severe or life-threatening chickenpox Chickenpox pneumonia	Dose for all ages 10 mg/kg 8-hourly by intravenous infusion over 1 hour; overdosage or more rapid infusion can cause raised blood urea; check blood count and blood urea
Vidarabine		Dose for all ages 10 mg/kg daily by intravenous infusion; check blood count
		In both cases reduce dose if there is renal impairment or falling blood count

16

Congenital and Perinatal Infections

Congenital infection

This occurs when a pathogen in the circulation of a pregnant woman crosses the placenta to infect the fetus. In the 40 weeks of her pregnancy a woman is very likely to suffer from one or more trivial infections but, fortunately, not many such conditions affect the fetus adversely. Chickenpox, for instance, can occur in pregnancy and, like any feverish condition, tends to hasten labour but even though the baby may be born with a rash or have serological evidence of recent infection, fetal damage is extremely rare. Even such diseases as influenza, hepatitis A and typhoid fever can occur during pregnancy without causing any defect in the infant.

Some congenital infections, however, are recognized as causing abortion, stillbirth, severe neonatal disease and sometimes fetal tissue damage with consequent developmental abnormalities. The best-known of these infections are Toxoplasmosis, Rubella, Cytomegalovirus infection and Herpes simplex (sometimes called the TORCH group of diseases). Syphilis and listeriosis can also cause fetal disease.

In general, the earlier in pregnancy the infection occurs, the more severe is the resulting fetal disease. Unfortunately the maternal infection is often mild and transient, or even subclinical, and often escapes notice.

Clinical signs

The response of the fetus to these severe, bloodborne infections is to develop multisystem disease. Fever may not be a major sign but a rash (often purpuric), thrombocytopenia, hepatitis, jaundice, encephalitis, pneumonitis and splenomegaly are all common. In addition each disease may produce its own features. Long-term effects, due to permanent tissue damage, can also occur and may become more marked as the child grows.

Diagnosis

The white blood cell count of the neonate is usually in the range of $18–25 \times 10^9/l$ with a marked neutrophilia. It is therefore not useful in the diagnosis of bacterial infection. Some authorities feel that the activated neutrophils of an infected baby will give a positive reaction in the Nitro-Blue Tetrazolium (NBT) test, but this investigation is not widely carried out.

Isolation of the pathogen from cord blood, urine or meconium provides a positive diagnosis.

Serological testing can be misleading, as a neonate may have acquired IgG antibodies transplacentally, and these often persist for weeks or months. Detection of IgM antibodies in cord blood, however, is evidence of recent fetal infection as IgM does not cross the placenta. High titres of IgG or other antibodies which do not fall in 2–6 months are unlikely to be maternally derived and also indicate infection of the fetus.

Perinatal infection

This follows exposure of the infant to a pathogen in the mother's genital tract during birth. The pathogen may either be infecting the genital tract or have migrated from its site in the bladder or the bowel. Maternal urinary tract or enteric infection is particularly likely to affect the infant if there is a long delay between rupture of the membranes and delivery. *Escherichia coli* and group B streptococci are the most common pathogens involved.

Perinatal infection may also be due to cytomegalovirus infection, listeriosis, herpes simplex, hepatitis B or enteric pathogens. There is usually a delay between delivery and the appearance of illness.

Clinical features and diagnosis
Although multisystem disease may occur, perinatal infection can be mild or even asymptomatic, depending mainly on the type of pathogen involved. There is no sign of infection at birth but when signs do appear some days or weeks later the diagnostic steps and treatment are exactly similar to those for congenital infection.

Toxoplasmosis

Origin of infection
Toxoplasmosis, due to the protozoan *Toxoplasma gondii* is a common infection in most communities, and particularly affects young adults. In Europe, between six and ten of every 1000 pregnant women acquire toxoplasmosis, while in Britain and the United States the rate is probably only two or three per 1000. A third to a half of infants born to infected mothers acquire congenital toxoplasmosis, and the risk is highest in the second half of the pregnancy. Only a half, or less, of infected infants have overt disease.

Clinical features
Approximately half of clinically affected infants are born with severe dis-

ease including rash, hepatosplenomegaly, meningoencephalitis and pneumonitis. Most also have chorioretinitis, the hallmark of congenital toxoplasmosis. Pale, fluffy retinal swellings on a reddened background later develop into white areas of denuded sclera surrounded by lacy black remnants of choroid tissue. These appearances persist into adulthood.

Long-term effects of severe infection include hydrocephaly, microcephaly, cerebral calcification, epilepsy, and mental and physical retardation.

Less severely affected infants are born with fever, abnormal liver function tests and choroiditis. Visual deficits may result from extensive or macular inflammation.

Diagnosis.
Two diagnostic findings are:

1. the presence of IgM complement-fixing antibodies to *T. gondii* in cord blood
2. toxoplasma dye test titre of 128 or greater in the infant's cerebrospinal fluid.

The infant usually has a serum dye test titre of greater than 1000, but this could be transplacentally derived.

T. gondii can be seen in, and cultured from, biopsy material but this is a tedious procedure and rarely carried out routinely.

Caution. Haemagglutinating antibodies may be undetectable in infants with congenital toxoplasmosis.

Treatment
It is too late to treat the infant once tissue damage has occurred. If the pregnant woman's infection is recognized she can be offered treatment with co-trimoxazole and/or pyrimethamine. These are both contraindicated, however, in early pregnancy. Therapeutic termination may then be offered, as fetal infection when it does occur in the first trimester is likely to be severe.

Rubella (German measles)

Origin of infection
Rubella is a common viral infection of children and young adults, whose incidence in many countries is changing now that immunization programmes have commenced. Infection in pregnancy is still not uncommon, however, and in the first 8 weeks of pregnancy transplacental infection occurs in about half of cases. Maternal infection in the third month will affect the fetus in one-third of cases but the consequences are less severe than in earlier infections. After the fifth month the risk of fetal damage is slight.

Clinical features

The range and severity of disorder is very wide varying from fetal death with abortion or stillbirth to permanent developmental abnormalities in a live child, or to mild problems such as low birthweight and slow development.

Temporary disorders.　These are the features of active fetal infection and include the familiar repertoire of anaemia, jaundice, hepatosplenomegaly, thrombocytopenia and meningoencephalitis. If the infant survives, these disorders resolve in the first 3 or 4 weeks of life.

Permanent disorders.　These result from permanent damage to developing tissues at the time of infection.

In the first month the brain, the eye and the heart are most severely affected. Cataracts are common, usually being dense and bilateral. Microphthalmia, chorioretinitis or glaucoma may also be seen. The most common cardiac defect is patent ductus arteriosus with or without pulmonary stenosis or septal defects. Mental and physical retardation are evident in most cases, becoming more noticeable as the child gets older.

In the second month cardiac abnormalities still occur, and damage to the inner ear can cause nerve deafness which may worsen over months or years.

Rarer manifestations.　These include osteochondritis of long bones, present at birth but resolving within about 6 months, thyroid dysfunction, early diabetes mellitus and a rare, progressive encephalopathy similar to subacute sclerosing panencephalitis (SSPE).

The expanded rubella syndrome.　This term was used to describe severe cases with both major and rare features of the disease, seen in a large epidemic during the 1960s. Osteochondritis was common in these infants.

Diagnosis

Identification of rubella virus in the faeces or urine of the infant confirms the diagnosis. Indirect confirmation of infection depends on the demonstration of IgM antibodies in cord blood.

Caution.　Affected infants may excrete rubella virus for many months after birth, a significant hazard to any susceptible pregnant women who are in contact with them.

Prevention

Immunization of girls and women before the commencement of

childbearing will prevent the occurrence of infection during pregnancy.

Human normal immunoglobulin in large doses may prevent the development of rubella in a susceptible person if given soon after exposure, but success is by no means guaranteed.

Termination of pregnancy may be offered to a woman who has acquired rubella during gestation.

Treatment
There is no effective treatment.

Cytomegalovirus (CMV)

Origin of infection
Neonatal cytomegalovirus infection can result from either transplacental, intrapartum or perinatal transfer of virus.

Congenital infection.
This is thought to occur in up to 2% of pregnancies worldwide. Most maternal infections are probably followed by fetal infection. Infection of the fetus in the first trimester tends to produce clinical disease, while progressively later infections are more likely to be subclinical.

Most congenital infections follow primary infection of the mother, but viraemia can recur during recrudescences of infection and some women are unlucky enough to have a second affected infant.

Perinatal infection. This is probably much more common than congenital infection, as 10% or more of women can be shown to excrete cytomegalovirus in genital secretions during late pregnancy. Some women also excrete virus in breast milk and may infect their infants by the oral route. Perinatal infection, however, seldom causes significant clinical illness.

Clinical features
The commonest clinical feature of congenital infection is low birth weight, though the severe picture of pneumonitis, jaundice, hepatosplenomegaly, encephalitis and thrombocytopenia is sometimes seen.

Early congenital infection can be followed by permanent disorders such as chorioretinitis, mental retardation, imperforate anus and cardiac abnormalities.

Diagnosis
Cytomegalovirus is detectable by standard tissue culture techniques, and is present in the urine of infected infants. It is present at birth after con-

genital infection, but appears after 2 or 3 weeks of life in perinatal infection.

Treatment and prophylaxis
No effective treatment or prophylaxis is available. Termination of pregnancy may be offered if maternal infection is detected.

Herpes simplex

Origin of infection
Herpes simplex viraemia may occur in a woman who has orofacial or genital infection. On the rare occasions when this occurs in pregnancy, transplacental infection of the fetus may result. The type of herpes virus involved will depend on the site of the mother's infection.

Perinatal infection is likely if a woman has genital herpes simplex at the time of delivery. In this case herpesvirus type 2 is the usual pathogen.

Clinical features
Congenital infection tends to produce severe systemic disease with encephalitis, pneumonitis, jaundice and a generalized rash, which may be vesicular or haemorrhagic or both.

Perinatal infection initially affects the oral, conjunctival and genital mucous membranes and the eye, though extension to the lungs and development of systemic disease is common.

In a recent study about half of affected infants had disseminated disease, a quarter had encephalitis alone, and the remainder had localized skin or mucous membrane infection.

Diagnosis
Herpesvirus is easily identifiable by standard tissue culture techniques and can be recovered from skin lesions, urine, CSF and biopsy material.

Typical skin lesions may permit a clinical diagnosis to be made at presentation, an important point as prompt treatment can significantly improve the prognosis.

Treatment
The antiviral drugs vidarabine and acyclovir are both effective against most herpesviruses. In systemic infection, however, tissue damage is severe and although treatment may reduce mortality, severe neurological sequelae are common. In localized infections treatment is often rapidly effective and it appears to prevent the later development of ocular or neurological disease.

Mortality in untreated systemic disease is about 80% and in encephalitis is about 30%

Syphilis

Origin of infection

A woman is most likely to transmit syphilis to her fetus if she becomes pregnant during the first year of her illness. In subsequent years congenital infection becomes both less likely and less severe. Transplacental spread of syphilis is rare before the fourth month of gestation, but can occur after this even if the mother is only infected very shortly before delivery.

Clinical features

Congenital syphilis early in the mother's disease commonly causes abortion or stillbirth. A severely affected infant may have systemic disorders similar to those seen in other congenital diseases.

Less severely affected infants often appear normal at birth, but develop symptoms soon after. Snuffles due to rhinitis may be overlooked, but jaundice and rash are also common. The rash is similar to that of adult secondary syphilis, often most noticeable on the palms, soles, face and perineum, and having a tendency to desquamate. At this stage osteochondritis of many bones is common, particularly of the face and lower limbs and leading eventually to 'saddle nose' and 'sabre shin'. Death in the first year is not uncommon, but, if the infant survives, the infection then becomes latent.

Late manifestations include notched upper incisors (Hutchinson's teeth), bossed permanent molars (mulberry molars), mandibular, palatal and cranial thickening, effusions into the knee joints (Clutton's joints), episodes of interstitial keratitis, and neurosyphilis. Nerve deafness is common.

Diagnosis

The early skin and mucous membrane lesions contain numerous spirochaetes which are detectable by dark-ground microscopy of scrapings. If this is not possible serological tests must be carried out at birth and after 6 weeks. If high titres of antibodies are maintained during this time, congenital infection is likely.

Prevention

If the mother's infection is detected and treated before the fourth month of pregnancy, fetal infection is unlikely to occur.

Treatment

Vigorous treatment of the mother may eradicate fetal infection during pregnancy, but follow-up of the infant is important, in case infection has merely become latent.

The infant should be treated as soon as the diagnosis is made. As with adults the drug of choice is one of the soluble penicillins, preferably benzylpenicillin for small babies. Full treatment should be offered, even if diagnosis is delayed to adolescence or adulthood as late manifestations, including neurosyphilis, may then be avoided.

Other sexually transmissible diseases

Ophthalmia neonatorum has been discussed in Chapter 2, but both gonococci and chlamydiae can cause other neonatal disease.

Gonococcal vulvovaginitis is an uncommon infection of female infants, contracted during birth.

Chlamydial infection can also be acquired during birth, usually when the mother has a history of vaginal discharge or pelvic disease during pregnancy. Chest infection is the common result and can present at any time up to 20 weeks after delivery, with rapid onset of respiratory distress but rarely with fever. The physical signs are those of bronchitis, bronchiolitis or pneumonitis. Treatment with erythromycin often produces improvement, but recovery is slow and relapse is not uncommon after treatment is stopped.

Hepatitis B can also be acquired at birth if the mother is suffering from active disease or is a HBeAg carrier. The infected infant will probably become a permanent carrier unless promptly given hyperimmune globulin (HBIG). Although the optimum regimen is not well established it is essential that the first dose of immunoglobulin is given within 48 hours, and that two to six further doses are given at monthly intervals.

Listeriosis

Origin of infection
This is a rare disease of the newborn which can occur either in a congenital form following maternal bacteraemia, or in a perinatal form associated with maternal genital infection.

Maternal infection can be acquired from a variety of sources, as *Listeria monocytogenes* is widely distributed in soil, vegetables and contaminated water. Bacteraemia in adults is often inapparent, though may be indicated by an influenza-like illness sometimes with arthralgia, loin pain and skin irritation.

Clinical features
Congenital infection.   This can occur from about 5 months of gestation onwards. Abortion or stillbirth is common. If the infant is born alive it has a grave systemic illness associated with abscesses, or sometimes granuloma formation in the liver, spleen and adrenal glands. The baby is not feverish, but has hepatosplenomegaly and a rash of livid papules, especially noticeable on the legs and feet. It may also have meningoencephalitis.

Perinatal infection. This takes the form of a septicaemia or meningitis appearing 4–6 weeks after birth. It appears no different from other severe neonatal bacteraemic diseases.

Diagnosis
If the clinical features suggest congenital listeriosis the diagnosis can be confirmed by demonstrating numerous Gram-positive rods in the meconium (which is normally bacteriologically sterile). The organism can also be recovered from blood cultures, though if care is not taken it can be dismissed as a diphtheroid.

Blood and CSF will contain *L. monocytogenes* when perinatal infection becomes evident.

Treatment
A combination of benzylpenicillin and erythromycin will eradicate the bacteraemia. Streptomycin and narrow-spectrum cephalosporins are also useful. Severe tissue damage, however, makes a favourable outcome difficult to achieve.

Prevention
If maternal bacteraemia or genital colonization is recognized, the mother may be treated with large doses of penicillin and erythromycin in an effort to prevent or curtail fetal disease.

Other neonatal bacterial infections

Origin of infection
The maternal genital tract can be colonized by a variety of organisms some of which, like group B streptococci, are resident flora while others are associated with disease in the mother. Common diseases which may affect a woman at the time of delivery include *Escherichia coli* urinary tract infections, and enteric infections due to such agents as salmonellae and *Campylobacter spp.* Group B streptococci are common colonists of the rectum and/or the genital tract, and are a common cause of neonatal disease.

A long interval between rupture of the membranes and the commencement of labour greatly increases the likelihood of fetal infection with contaminating organisms. The result of fetal infection is often a neonatal bacteraemia or meningitis presenting 2 or 3 days after birth. Later infections, presenting at age 3 or 4 weeks, are also seen.

Diagnosis
If an infant collapses or has a severe feverish illness during the neonatal period, cultures should be taken from both the infant and the mother. Blood, stool, urine and CSF should be obtained from the infant while

urine, stool and vaginal samples are taken from the mother. The infant's and the mother's organisms are often the same.

Treatment

As with bacteraemic disease in adults, treatment should be begun as soon as adequate samples have been obtained for bacteriological studies. Group B streptococcal infection can be expected to respond to treatment with benzylpenicillin, cephalosporins, erythromycin, or high-dose ampicillin or amoxycillin. Gram-negative infections are usually treated with aminoglycosides such as gentamicin or kanamycin which may be combined with very wide-spectrum penicillins or cephalosporins (see Chapter 10).

In salmonella infections, although other agents often appear to be effective *in vitro*, chloramphenicol alone may affect the disease in the clinical setting. If it must be used, it should be given in small doses, as the immature liver of the neonate cannot detoxify it and a shock syndrome (grey baby syndrome) can easily be precipitated by overdosage.

Prevention

If the mother's infection is amenable to antibiotic therapy, it should be adequately treated before delivery.

A delay of more than 48 hours between rupture of the membranes and delivery should be avoided if possible.

Babies born of infected mothers should be carefully followed up in the neonatal period.

Unfortunately, prophylactic antibiotic treatment of the newborn has not always proved effective in preventing neonatal infection. Many paediatricians would give penicillin and gentamicin to a neonate whose mother had significant fever during delivery, and there is evidence that this prevents some severe perinatal disease.

Drugs mentioned in this chapter

Drug	Indication	Usage and precautions
Acyclovir	Neonatal herpes simplex infections	Local infection: dose is 5 mg/kg 8-hourly by intravenous infusion over 1 hour; systemic infection: dose is double; check blood urea and blood count
Benzylpenicillin	Maternal listeriosis or syphilis	Dose is 1.2–2.4 g (2–4 mega units) 6-hourly, intravenously continued for 10–14 days (significant amounts will cross the placenta and may help to eradicate fetal infection)

	Neonatal infections	Dose is 50–200 mg/kg daily, in divided doses intravenously
Co-trimoxazole	Maternal toxoplasmosis	Dose is 960 mg 8–12-hourly, orally, for 2 weeks
Erythromycin	Maternal listeriosis	Dose 2.0–4.0 g daily in divided doses, intravenously
	Neonatal infections	Dose is 30–50 mg/kg daily intravenously, in four divided doses
Gentamicin	Neonatal Gram-negative infections	Infant dose: 6 mg/kg daily in divided doses: up to 2 weeks old in two 12-hourly doses; over age 2 weeks in three 8-hourly doses, check peak and trough levels
	Intrathecal dosage	1 mg daily intrathecally with 2.0–4.0 mg/kg daily intramuscularly in divided doses
Vidabarin	Alternative to acyclovir	Dose for all ages 10 mg/kg daily by intravenous infusion; check blood count; usual course is 5 days, but may be given for longer

17

Imported Diseases

Introduction

Wherever in the world a physician works there is always the chance that a visitor will import an unfamiliar disease which is not endemic to the area. Such diseases always cause concern because clinical suspicion of them is low, facilities for diagnosis may be limited, and knowledge of treatment and complications may be incomplete.

A huge expansion in air travel during the last two decades has contributed largely to the problem of imported disease (Fig. 23 a and b),

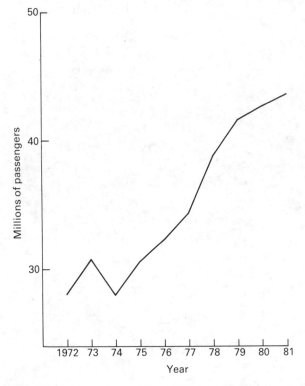

Fig. 23a. Increase in air travel to and from UK since 1972 (figures from CAA statistics unit).

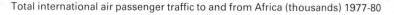

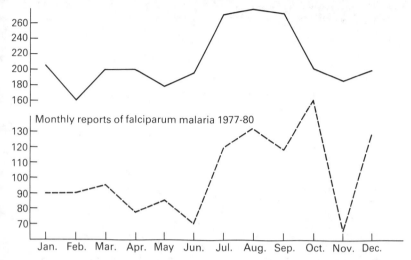

Total international air passenger traffic to and from Africa (thousands) 1977-80

Monthly reports of falciparum malaria 1977-80

Fig. 23b. Reports of falciparum malaria and air travel to and from Africa (CDSC).

indeed most air journeys can be accomplished in a time which is shorter than the incubation periods of most diseases.

Not only the country from which the traveller arrives, but the part of the country is important. Large countries may possess a variety of terrains including jungle, swamp, grassland and desert, all of which will harbour different pathogens and disease vectors. Exposure as brief as the entry of a mosquito through a vehicle door or the drinking of a glass of water may be followed by significant illness.

Management of a traveller with feverish illness

Types of disease to consider
Worldwide 'cosmopolitan' diseases. These are common causes of fever in most countries and are as likely to be imported as indigenous. They include:

influenza
urinary infections
childhood diseases
infectious mononucleosis
sexually transmitted diseases

viral infections
pneumonias
tuberculosis
septicaemias

It is worth remembering that the antibiotic sensitivities of imported bacterial infections may differ somewhat from those of the local flora.

Staphylococci and gonococci are particular examples of this, for methicillin-resistant staphylococci are common in the Middle East, and penicillin-resistant gonococci are common in the Far East and Indonesia.

Diseases controllable by public health measures. 'Westernized' countries enjoy such public health facilities as safe water supplies, effective sanitation, and immunization programmes against infectious diseases. In countries without such facilities enteric pathogens often contaminate water and are transferred to salads and fruit by washing and to drinks in ice cubes. Epidemic diseases may also occur; these include:

salmonellosis	cholera
amoebic dysentery	bacillary dysentery
diphtheria	poliomyelitis
enteric fevers	infectious hepatitis
giardiasis	

Diseases with a restricted distribution. The restricted distribution is usually due to environmental requirements of the pathogen or its vector. A good example is the parasite of malaria which can only reproduce in the mosquito when the environmental temperature is sufficiently high; such diseases include:

malaria	viral haemorrhagic fevers
yellow fever	

Diseases acquired from animals. Travellers may come into contact with unusual animals, or with infected animals, by several means. They may be bitten, licked or scratched by the animal. They may come into contact with its carcase or hide. They may drink its milk or eat its cheese and yoghurt. They may even share its stable or byre and be bitten by its parasites; diseases include:

rabies	plague (rare)
rickettsioses	Q fever
brucellosis	ornithosis

Travellers at special risk
These are people who have been abroad to work and have suffered occupational exposure to particular terrains, disease vectors, animals or sick people. They include:

site engineers	missionaries
nurses	illegal immigrants
refugees	doctors
land surveyors	disaster relief workers

Points to emphasize in history-taking

Places visited and dates of visits. The importance of obtaining an accurate travel history cannot be overemphasized, for much anxiety and delay can be avoided by this means. A person visiting an industrial city, or tropical jungle, for instance, will not have been exposed to viral haemorrhagic fever, but may have contracted malaria. A trip to the Mediterranean will carry little risk of malaria, but enteric fever is a significant possibility in several areas. It is important to ask the patient what type of countryside was encountered, whether insects or rodents were a problem, where the water supply was obtained and how satisfactory were sanitary services.

The dates of visits are of paramount importance, particularly dates of entry to, and exit from, known endemic areas, for these must be compared with the incubation periods of various possible diseases.

Means and routes of travel. Those who travel overland are more likely to be exposed to disease than those who go by air. Camping, drinking stream water and bathing in fresh water are common hazards to which overland travellers are exposed.

Stopovers on air or sea journeys may be times of specific risk, for instance by insect bite, exposure to contaminated food or water or by sexual exposure. Many travellers also make small excursions or day trips 'out of town' or 'up country' which they may forget unless specifically questioned.

Prophylaxis and precautions taken. Travellers vary greatly in the preparations which they make for their journey, and may have difficulty in obtaining accurate advice. Any vaccinations as well as the nature of malarial prophylaxis and the care with which it is taken should be noted. It should be remembered, however, that no immunization is completely effective in every case, and that malarial prophylaxis may be inadequate after forgetting tablets, following gastrointestinal disorders, if medication is discontinued too soon after leaving the endemic area, and in areas of drug resistance.

Clinical assessment

Unfortunately many imported diseases have rather indeterminate clinical features in the early stages, and diagnosis must rest on a high index of suspicion and a repeated search for helpful clinical features. Such features include:

1. Abdominal distension and rose spots in enteric fevers.
2. Rash and conjunctival suffusion in rickettsioses.
3. Extremely severe headache in rickettisioses.
4. Myalgia in leptospirosis and rickettsioses.

5. Jaundice; with bilirubinuria in hepatitis, and without bilirubinuria in malaria.
6. Fever; with stepladder increase in enteric fever, becoming intermittent in malaria.

Laboratory investigations
These are essentially the same as for the investigation of any fever (see Chapter 18). Two important common diseases, however, must not be missed as they can be fatal if not promptly treated. They are malaria and enteric fever, both of which are easily initially dismissed as 'severe influenza'. Blood films for malarial parasites and blood cultures for salmonellae should be *repeatedly* examined until a diagnosis is satisfactorily established.

Malaria

Epidemiology
This is a disease caused by protozoa of the genus *Plasmodium*. It is widely distributed in tropical areas where it is an important cause of morbidity and mortality. The sexual cycle of the parasite takes place in the gut of an *Anopheles sp.* mosquito and the resulting sporozoites migrate to the salivary glands from which they are injected into a human when the mosquito bites. Asexual forms then develop in the liver before invading red blood cells and appearing in the circulation. Eventually gametocytes form in the erythrocytes, and can complete the lifecycle if ingested by a biting mosquito (Fig. 24).

The mosquito lays its eggs on the surface of still water and its larvae and pupae are aquatic. Ponds, puddles, tanks and cisterns in hot climates are the breeding grounds for the insect vector on which the disease depends.

Four types of plasmodia infect humans: *P. vivax*, *P. falciparum*, *P. malariae* and *P. ovale*. Vivax malaria is much the commonest type in the Indian subcontinent, while falciparum malaria predominates in Africa, Indonesia and parts of South America (Fig. 25 *see* p. 230). *P. falciparum* is the cause of malignant tertian malaria; the other plasmodia cause benign tertian and quartan malarias.

Clinical features
Acute infections.   The incubation period is usually 10–14 days, but can be up to 6 weeks in malariae malaria. The parasites then invade the red cells and multiply. The infected erythrocytes are eventually destroyed as the parasites are released to invade further cells. The release of parasites is associated with episodes of rigors, high fever and sweating which last for several hours. Initially the fever is chaotic, but after several days, release of parasites becomes synchronized and the fever becomes intermittent. In vivax and ovale infections the fever is *tertian*, appearing on

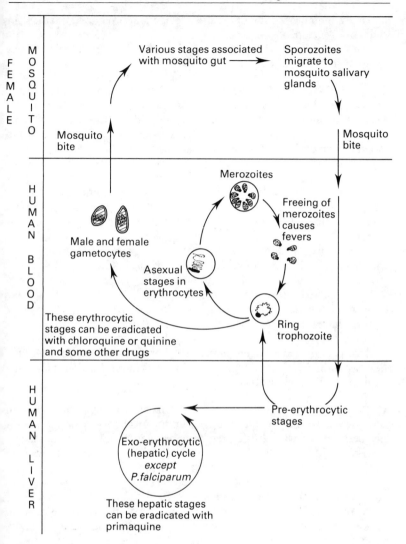

Fig. 24. Lifecycle of malarial parasites.

every first and third day. In malariae infections it is *quartan*, appearing on every first and fourth day. In falciparum malaria synchronization is less complete, but may produce a tertian pattern.

Anaemia is common, partly due to direct destruction of red blood cells and partly to an immune response to parasitized cells. In falciparum malaria a high proportion of cells is affected and profound anaemia can suddenly develop.

The spleen is modestly enlarged, and appears as a firm palpable mass in more than half of patients.

Malignant (falciparum) malaria.   This is the severe disease caused by *P. falciparum* infection. In individuals with no immunity at all it can be fulminating and fatal. In apparently immune residents of endemic areas it can appear 10–14 days after arrival in a cooler climate. Its main effects are severe haemolysis, cerebral damage and renal damage.

Haemolysis can be sudden and life-threatening, producing haemoglobinaemia and haemoglobinuria (the features of blackwater fever).

Cerebral malaria is due to a mixture of cerebral oedema, occlusion of small blood vessels by sludging of red cells, and vascular damage leading to haemorrhage. It produces drowsiness, convulsions and coma, and can be rapidly fatal.

Renal damage is due to a mixture of sludging and vascular damage in the renal circulation, combined with tubular damage after haemoglobinuria. Acute renal failure can occur.

Disseminated intravascular coagulation (DIC) can occur if vascular damage is widespread. The anaemia is then exacerbated by haemorrhage.

Pulmonary oedema is a rare feature of malignant malaria.

If the patient survives the acute attack, immune mechanisms may produce a continuing fall in the haemoglobin level or platelet count for some days or weeks afterwards.

Chronic and recurrent malaria.   In patients with 'benign' malarias who have overcome the parasitaemia by immune mechanisms, or in whom it has been treated with drugs, there may be relapses of fever at increasing intervals. This is because *P. vivax*, *P. ovale* and *P. malariae* can persist in the liver and periodically reinvade the red blood cells. Without treatment, relapses gradually cease within about 2 years except in *P. malariae* infections which may persist for much longer.

People who have frequent relapses and reinfections tend to develop chronic anaemia, massive friable enlargement of the spleen and, rarely, immune complex glomerulonephritis.

Caution.   Although residents in endemic areas develop a degree of immunity to malaria this is rapidly lost on leaving the area. After 2 years all immunity is lost and malarial prophylaxis is *essential* if the endemic area is revisited.

Diagnosis
The white cell count may be normal or raised.

The finding of parasites in the red blood cells is diagnostic. Thick and thin blood films are examined; these may be made at the bedside or from an anticoagulated blood sample for blood cell examination.

Caution. Repeated blood examinations may be necessary. Inadequate prophylaxis or recent treatment with sulphonamides will partially eradicate the parasitaemia, making initial diagnosis very difficult.

Serology. An immunofluorescent antibody test is available. A positive test indicates recent, though not necessarily current, infection.

Treatment
Treatment of acute infections. This treatment should eradicate the erythrocyte stages of the parasite, and is all that is required in falciparum infections.

The treatment of choice is chloroquine, which is usually given orally, but may be given by injection in severely ill patients.

If chloroquine-resistant falciparum malaria is suspected, or if the patient is extremely ill, quinine is the drug of choice. If it is being used to treat cerebral malaria, it should always be given by intravenous infusion, with close observation in case of cardiac dysrrhythmias.

Fansidar® may also be used to treat chloroquine-resistant falciparum malaria, but it has a slow onset of activity and should not, therefore, be used alone.

Caution. Corticosteroids can be used to treat the cerebral oedema of falciparum malaria, but may possibly reduce the entry of antimalarial drugs into the brain. It is probably best to give corticosteroids *after* the first dose of antimalarials.

Eradication of hepatic parasites. Primaquine is the only drug available for this purpose. It has the disadvantage of causing haemolysis in individuals with glucose-6-phosphate dehydrogenase deficiency. G6PD activity should be estimated before treatment and the drug withheld if there is significant deficiency. Relapses in G6PD-deficient individuals must then be treated with chloroquine, as in acute infection, until they eventually cease.

Malarial prophylaxis
Visitors to endemic areas should take chemoprophylaxis (Table 9). Malaria in pregnancy is a dangerous disease; chemoprophylaxis is *not* contraindicated during pregnancy, though some precautions are advisable in the use of drugs.

Wearing clothes which cover the extremities, using insect repellent creams, mosquito nets and screens, and staying indoors at dusk will minimize exposure to infected mosquitoes.

Table 9.   Recommended chemoprophylaxis of malaria

All areas If *P. falciparum* anticipated	Proguanil (Paludrine) 200 mg daily, or chloroquine 300 mg (of base) weekly

If chloroquine-resistant
P. falciparum exists
	Maloprim (pyrimethamine + dapsone) one tablet
	weekly.
	or
	Fansidar (pyrimethamine + sulphadoxine) one
	tablet weekly.
	NB These drugs are not recommended in early
	    pregnancy. Chloroquine will prevent most attacks;
	    others may be treated with quinine.

Children
   Up to 1 year
   1–5 years
   6–12 years
	
	One-quarter of adult dose
	Half adult dose
	Three-quarters adult dose

Rickettsial infections

Epidemiology
Rickettsiae are natural pathogens of small animals and are transmitted to man by arthropod vectors. Human infection usually follows close contact with either the arthropods or the small animals themselves. An exception to this scheme is epidemic typhus, whose cycle is between man and the human body louse (Table 10).

Clinical features
Epidemic typhus and Rocky Mountain spotted fever (RMSF) are severe diseases. The others may be debilitating, but are rarely fatal.

Most patients with the two severe diseases recall prolonged contact with the arthropod vector. The incubation period is 7–10 days, longest in epidemic typhus.

Illness begins abruptly and the major features are very high fever, severe headache and myalgia, and rash which begins on the fourth or fifth day. In RMSF the rash is maculopapular and spreads from the extremities to the trunk; in typhus it is macular and spreads from the axillae to the trunk and upper limbs. A petechial element is common and haemorrhages or ecchymoses appear in severe cases.

Rigors, conjunctival redness, constipation, abnormal liver function tests and rising blood urea are commonly seen. In fatal cases uraemia, haemorrhage, sludging of red blood cells and thromboses are the usual cause of death.

Table 10. Rickettsioses

Disease	Organism	Transmission	Weil–Felix
RMSF	R. rickettsii	Tick bite	
Boutonneuse fever	R. conorii	Tick bite	⎧ OX-19
Queensland tick			⎨ and
typhus	R. australis	Tick bite	⎩ OX-2
N. Asian tick			
typhus	R. siberica	Tick bite	
Scrub typhus	R. tsutsugamushi	Mite bite	OX-K
Rickettsialpox	R. akari	Mite bite	Negative
Trench fever	R. quintana	Inoculation of	Negative
Epidemic typhus	R. prowazekii	infected louse faeces	OX-19
Endemic (murine) typhus	R. mooseri	Flea bite	OX-19

Diagnosis
There is usually a neutrophil leukocytosis.

The Weil–Felix reaction. This is a non-specific agglutination by the patient's serum of certain *Proteus spp.* OX antigens. It is a useful screening test for groups of rickettsioses.

Specific complement-fixation tests. Complement-fixing antibodies appear early in the course of the disease, and a significant rising titre in paired sera is good evidence of the specific infection.

Identification of organism. Rickettsiae may be seen in histological preparations of skin and lymph node biopsy. They can be isolated from tissues in specially equipped laboratories.

Caution. The petechial rash can be mistaken for that of meningococcal disease. If there is doubt both disorders should be treated while the diagnosis is ascertained.
   The rash of rickettsialpox has a vesicular element, but the presence also of macular and nodular lesions helps to distinguish it from chickenpox.
   Epidemic typhus may recur many years after an original infection (Brill–Zinsser disease). In such recurrences the Weil–Felix reaction is usually negative, but specific complement-fixing antibodies quickly reappear.

Treatment
All of the rickettsioses respond to treatment with tetracyclines.

Chloramphenicol is also effective. The drugs can usually be given orally.

Arbovirus infections

Epidemiology
Arboviruses naturally exist in birds and small animals. They are transmitted by the bite of arthropods such as mosquitoes, sandflies, ticks and mites. Both farm animals and humans can become infected.

Clinical features
Most arbovirus infections are acute and severe, but they are almost always self-limiting and have negligible mortality. Characteristic features are as follows (Table 11).

Short incubation periods.   Usually 3–7 days.

Abrupt onset.   Fever, headache, myalgia, reddened conjunctivae and enanthem of tiny vesicles on the palate.

Tendency to temporary improvement.   A brief fall in temperature after 3 or 4 days gives the temperature chart a 'saddleback' appearance.

Neutropenia.   When the fever is established the white blood cell count is often below $4 \times 10^9/l$.

Additional features.   These are mentioned in Table 11 opposite.

Diagnosis
This is usually only possible if virus can be isolated from blood or pharyngeal washings in the first days of illness. Antibodies to dengue viruses are detectable in serum, but false-positive results are common after yellow fever immunization.

Treatment
This is symptomatic. Rare cases of haemorrhagic disease may need intensive care, and it should be remembered that the patient's blood and body fluids may be infectious.

Viral haemorrhagic fevers

Epidemiology
These are systemic viral infections which have a rather limited distribution in the world (Table 12). They occasionally cause local epidemics, or sporadic infections in visitors to the endemic areas, and at these times mortality is often very high.

Table 11. Arbovirus infections

Disease	Vector	Distribution
Feverish illness with headache and myalgia		
Phlebotomus fever	Sandfly	East Africa, Eastern Mediterranean, Central Asia
Colorado tick fever	Tick	Colorado Valley
Rift Valley fever	Mosquito	African Rift Valley
Plus maculopapular rash and large-joint arthralgia		
Chikungunya fever	}	Africa, India, Eastern Asia
Mayaro fever	Mosquito	Caribbean, Brazil
Sindbis fever		Eastern Africa
O nyong-nyong fever		Africa, India, Eastern Asia, Australia
Plus rash, which may desquamate, and lymphadenopathy including occipital and epitrochlear nodes		
Dengue fevers (types 1 to 4)	Mosquito	Various types throughout the tropical world
West Nile fever		Africa, Eastern Europe, India, Indonesia
Rare association with haemorrhagic rash and high mortality		
Dengue haemorrhagic fever	Mosquito	See above
Chikungunya haemorrhagic fever		See above
Yellow fever		Tropical Africa, Central and South America

It is likely that all are transmitted by small animals which excrete the virus in their urine. In the case of Lassa fever the animal is the multi-mammate rat *Mastomys natalensis*. Natural infection can be acquired when a rat urinates upon its human captors or when human skin is penetrated by urine-soaked vegetation.

Table 12. Viral haemorrhagic fevers

Haemorrhagic fever	Virus	Distribution
Lassa fever	Lassa	East Africa, especially Nigeria, Liberia, Sierra Leone
Argentinian haemorrhagic fever	Junin	Argentina
Bolivian haemorrhagic fever	Machupo	Bolivia
Marburg haemorrhagic fever	Marburg	Central and tropical South Africa
Ebola haemorrhagic fever	Ebola	Central Africa
Congo-Crimean haemorrhagic fever	Unknown	Central Africa, Eastern Europe, Near East
Korean haemorrhagic fever	? Hantan	Korea, Northern Europe, USSR

Person-to-person spread is relatively rare, as the viruses are only briefly present on the skin or in pharyngeal secretions. Sick-bed attendants are at risk, however, as virus is present in the patient's body fluids and, later, in the urine. Inoculation or ingestion accidents can infect medical and laboratory staff.

Clinical features
The incubation period is usually 10–14 days, and is taken not to be more than 20 days. Symptoms are entirely non-specific, usually being gradual onset of fever, anorexia, myalgia and vomiting. They cannot be distinguished from the early features of malaria, viral hepatitis or enteric fevers. Often the patient becomes more and more ill until multisystem failure leads to uraemia and haemorrhagic manifestations. The few patients who have been investigated show evidence of bone marrow, liver, kidney and muscle damage. The patient remains orientated until the terminal stages.

Helpful features in Lassa fever include pharyngitis with white patchy exudate, abdominal tenderness and non-pitting oedema of the face and neck. In Marburg and Ebola disease a maculopapular rash, diarrhoea and exudative pharyngitis tend to appear in the first week. In Korean haemorrhagic fever glomerulonephritis is often seen.

Diagnosis
The agents of viral haemorrhagic fevers (VHF) are classed as dangerous, or category A pathogens and must not be handled in routine laboratories. A very detailed history of travel should be taken, covering the last 3 weeks before illness. If the epidemiological or clinical features suggest VHF, expert advice should be sought.

Caution. The patient must not be allowed to succumb to a much commoner disease, such as malaria, while the question of VHF is under investigation. If his condition causes concern, chloroquine should be given. Chloramphenicol is a useful broad-spectrum drug if other diseases are also causing serious concern. It has the advantage of not requiring injection.

Arranging safe management
Do not send blood or other samples to local laboratories.
Consult the local infectious diseases specialist.
Inform the responsible Medical Officer of Environmental Health (MOEH)
Detailed information may then be obtained from the sources listed at the end of this chapter. The MOEH is usually responsible for collecting information. Arrangements will be made for high-security transport and management of the patient, and examination of specimens. This is usually done by the MOEH and the infectious diseases specialist.

Health precautions when travelling abroad

Begin planning in good time before departure
This is because primary immunization for some diseases requires one month between doses. The absolute minimum time between successive doses is 2 weeks, but this is at the cost of reduced protection.

A yellow fever vaccination certificate does not become valid until 10 days after a first immunization.

Comply with International Health Regulations (IHR)
Many countries in Africa and Central and South America cannot be entered without a valid International Certificate of Yellow Fever vaccination.

Countries where cholera is endemic may from time to time require a certificate of immunization against cholera. Travel agents are aware of current IHR requirements, but may not be so well-informed about other advisable precautions.

Prepare to take malarial prophylaxis. The appropriate drugs are readily available from chemists. Some can cause troublesome side-effects, so it is worthwhile taking a test dose 2 or 3 weeks before departure. This allows time to change if necessary. Obtain enough tablets for the whole visit if possible, as they may not be readily available at the destination.

Consider typhoid immunization. The best protection against enteric infections is strict personal hygiene. There is no immunization available against paratyphoid fevers, but monovalent typhoid vaccine is effective. It is worth being immunized or having a booster dose if travelling to tropical or hot areas.

Remember poliomyelitis. If typhoid immunization is worthwhile, so probably is poliomyelitis immunization, or a booster dose.

Protection against hepatitis A. This is indicated for people who go to work in areas where sanitation or safe water supply is unreliable. Many adults are already immune and possess IgG antiHAV. Otherwise human normal immunoglobulin (HIG) may be given (see Chapter 20).

Remember rabies. Do not approach animals unnecessarily. Act promptly if bitten or scratched (see Chapter 9).

Sources of information on imported diseases

Specialist information

United Kingdom.
   1. International Relations Division,

Department of Health and Social Security,
Alexander Flemming House, Elephant and Castle,
London, SE1 6BY (01 407 5522)
2. Scottish Home and Health Department,
St Andrew's House,
Edinburgh, EH1 3DE (031 556 8501)
3. Department of Health and Social Services,
Dundonald House, Upper Newtownards Road,
Belfast, BJ4 3SF (0232 63939)
4. Welsh Office, Cathays Park,
Cardiff, CF1 3NQ (0222 825111)

General.
Epidemiological Surveillance of Communicable Diseases,
World Health Organization, 1211 Geneva 27, Switzerland
Telegraph: EPIDNATIONS, GENEVA.

Information for travellers
1. *Notice to Travellers: Protect Your Health Abroad.* Department of
Health and Social Security leaflet SA35.
Available from: Travel Agents
or Social Security offices
or DHSS Leaflets Unit, PO Box 21,
Stanmore, Middlesex, HA7 1AY
2. *Vaccination Certificate Requirements for International Travel and
Health Advice to Travellers.* Published by the World Health
Organization, Geneva.
Available from: Her Majesty's Stationery Office,
49 High Holborn, London, WC1V 6HB
and other branches of HMSO
or WHO Distribution and Sales Service,
1211 Geneva 27, Switzerland

Drugs mentioned in this chapter

Drug	Indication	Usage and precautions
Chloramphenicol	Rickettsioses: alternative to tetracycline	Adult dose 2.0–3.0 g daily in three or four divided doses orally or intravenously; child's dose is 50–100 mg/kg daily in divided doses; bone marrow depression occurs rarely; a continuing fall in the white cell count is an indication to stop dosage

Table 13.   Health risks to travellers

Distribution	Eastern Europe	Mediterranean	Asia	India	North and Central Africa	Central America and Panama Caribbean	South America	Australasia	Pacific	Indonesia
Transmission										
Food and water										
Hepatitis A*		+	+	+	+	+	+		+	+
Giardiasis		+	+	+	+	+	+		+	+
Enteric fever*		+	+	+	+	+	±		+	+
Cholera*C			+	+	±					+
Bacillary dysentery		+	+	+	+	+	+		+	+
Amoebic dysentery			+	+	+	+	+			+
Poliomyelitis*			+	+	+	+	±	+		+
Water contact										
Leptospirosis	+	+	+	+	+		+			+
Schistosomiasis		+			++	±	+			+
Arthropod spread										
Dengue fevers			+		+	±	±	+	+	+
Rickettsioses	+		+	+	+			+		+
Yellow fever*C					+	±	+			
Animal contact										
Brucellosis	+	+	±	+	+	+				
Rabies*	+	+	++	++	+	+	±	None		+

Immunization: *available; *C may be compulsory

NOTE   No indication means no great risk, *not* that the disease cannot be contracted

Chloroquine	Acute malaria including malignant malaria due to sensitive *P. falciparum*	Adult dose (as chloroquine base) 600 mg orally, followed by 300 mg after 6 hours, then 300 mg daily for two more days; if parenteral treatment is needed dose is chloroquine sulphate 200–300 mg by slow intravenous injection (intramuscular injection may act too slowly in a gravely ill or shocked patient); child's dose is a quarter to half of the adult dose; intravenous medication is contra-indicated in infants as dangerous cardiac dysrhythmias can occur.

	Malarial prophylaxis	For dose see Table 9; side-effects including disabling pruritis in dark-skinned races, nausea, vomiting, rare psychoses; prolonged dosage carries a small risk of visual impairment: colour vision should be checked 6-monthly
Fansidar (pyrimethamine plus sulphadoxine)	Prophylaxis of chloroquine-resistant malaria,	For dose see Table 9; side-effects include pyrimethamine allergy, sulphonamide allergy and rare bone marrow depression
	Acute chloroquine-resistant malaria	Adult dose three tablets immediately, orally; should not be given alone as onset of action is slow; one or two doses of an additional drug, such as quinine, should also be given
Maloprim (pyrimethamine plus dapsone)	Prophylaxis of chloroquine-resistant malaria	For dose see Table 9; side-effects include rashes and rare bone marrow depression
Primaquine	Eradication of hepatic cycle of benign malarias	Adult dose 15 mg daily, orally for 2 weeks; child's dose is 7.5 mg daily; contraindicated in G6PD deficiency
Proguanil	Malarial prophylaxis	For dose see Table 9; side-effects include epigastric discomfort and rare haematuria
Quinine (If quinine is unavailable quinidine 10 mg/kg may be given orally or by nasogastric tube until the correct medication can be used)	Acute chloroquine-resistant malaria and cerebral malaria	Adult dose 600 mg 8-hourly, orally for at least four doses; child's dose 5–10 mg/kg 8-hourly. In malignant or cerebral malaria when emergency treament is *essential*, adult dose 5–10 mg/kg as intravenous infusion over 4 hours; infants should be given 5 mg/kg intramuscularly to avoid dangerous cardiac dysrhythmias; side-effects include nausea, tinnitus, vertigo, deafness and cardiac dysrhythmias; the dose may have to be reduced if they occur; total infused should not be more than 500 mg per dose; four doses should be given at intervals of 12–24 hours.

| Tetracycline | Rickettsioses | Adult dose as oxytetracycline 500 mg 6-hourly, orally, continued for 7 days; child's dose is 50–100 mg/kg daily in four divided doses (may stain teeth); may be given intravenously in severe cases |

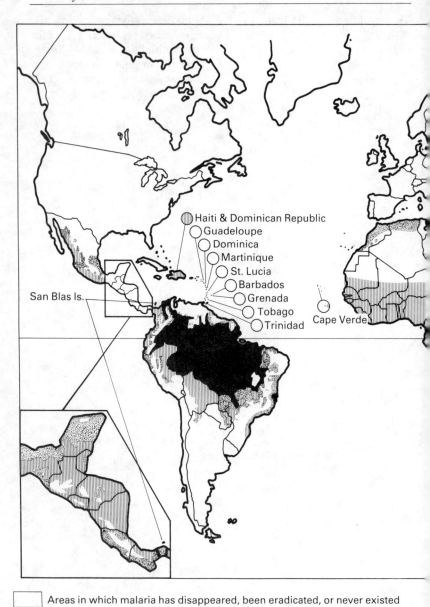

Areas in which malaria has disappeared, been eradicated, or never existed

Areas with limited risk

Fig. 25.   Epidemiological assessment of malaria in the world up to June 1982 (Malaria Reference Laboratory).

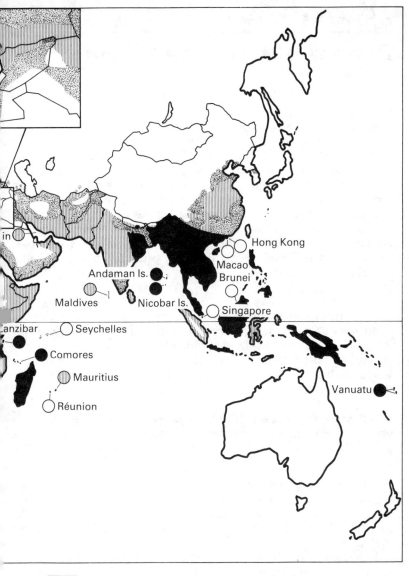

Hong Kong
Macao
Brunei
Andaman Is.
Maldives
Nicobar Is.
Singapore
anzibar · Seychelles
Comores
Mauritius
Réunion
Vanuatu

░░ Areas where malaria transmission occurs or might occur

■ *P.falciparum* resistant to chloroquine

18

Pyrexia of Unknown Origin

Introduction
Pyrexia of unknown origin (PUO) is the term used to describe a fever for which no cause is found after a period of investigation.

Of the whole range of feverish illnesses, transient viral infections are by far the most common and these seldom present to medical attention. Disorders which do present to medical attention often have distinct symptoms and signs which lead to the diagnosis within a few days. Some diseases, however, present with unusual features or with fever alone. In such cases it may take many days for the evolution of the illness or for a diagnostic test to solve the riddle of diagnosis. Most physicians would consider such an illness to be a PUO if it persisted undiagnosed after 3 weeks.

Causes of pyrexia of unknown origin
Several investigators have collected large series of cases of PUO, so that useful information is available about the common causes. Because many infectious diseases are self-limiting within 1 or 2 weeks they do not figure largely in the list. Infections which tend to be chronic, or for which there is an underlying surgical or medical cause are, however, among the commonest causes.

Infection: 30–40% of cases. PUO is an unusual presentation of a variety of infections. Diagnostic difficulty is due more often to obscurity of the site of infection than of the infection itself. Infections which are often causes of PUO are listed in approximate order of frequency:

1. pyogenic infection; abscesses of peritoneal reflections, liver, kidney, pancreas; osteomyelitis; sinusitis; dental sepsis.
2. urinary and biliary tract infections; these are often secondary to stone or stricture; absence of the expected symptoms and signs does not exclude the diagnosis.
3. tuberculosis; this is a common chronic disease throughout the world; non-pulmonary tuberculosis can be very difficult to diagnose.
4. subacute bacterial endocarditis; this is a rare disease which should always be sought as a cause of PUO, for delay in treatment can seriously affect the prognosis.
5. chronic or relapsing infections; this group includes prolonged illness due to infectious mononucleosis, cytomegalovirus infection, brucellosis, Q fever and toxoplasmosis.

Caution. Some infections may be prolonged or atypical because of underlying disorders. Examples include tuberculosis with underlying Hodgkin's disease, cytomegalovirus infection with underlying lymphocytic leukaemia and pyogenic infections with underlying granulocytic leukaemia.

Neoplasia: 20–30% of cases. Hodgkin's disease is the most common of fever-producing neoplasms. The classical, undulating Pel–Ebstein fever is seen less often than a low-grade, irregular fever.

Other tumours recognized as causes of PUO include non-Hodgkin's lymphomas, leukaemias, hypernephroma, hepatoma and the rare atrial myxoma.

Immunological disorders: 12–20% of cases. Drug reactions account for the largest part of this group. Drug fever is swinging and persistent, often low-grade but sometimes verging on hyperpyrexia. It may occur alone but association with rash, jaundice or blood disorder is common. In some cases drug reactions occur in patients who have been taking the same drug for months or years without previous difficulty. Common causes of drug reactions include aspirin, other salicylates, antibiotics, barbiturates, methyldopa, nitrofurantoin, phenytoin, procainamide, quinidine, hydralazine and antituberculosis agents.

Autoimmune and collagen diseases form the other major part of this group, and can cause confusion if they appear to be precipitated by an infectious disease or drug reaction. In adults systemic lupus erythematosus, polymyalgia rheumatica and polyarteritis nodosa may all present as PUO. In children Still's disease and dermatomyositis can produce the same picture. Rheumatic fever is another disorder which causes diagnostic difficulty if its presentation is atypical.

Other causes. These, of course, are numerous but granulomatous disorders such as sarcoidosis and Crohn's disease are common and therefore high on the list. Rare diseases of unknown aetiology such as familial Mediterranean fever and Mollaret's meningitis also fall into this group.

Undiagnosed: 5–25% of cases. In many cases the fever gradually subsides over a period of weeks or months. A few patients have persisting or recurring fever which is low-grade and often associated with episodes of mild to moderate malaise.

Investigation of pyrexia of unknown origin

This is no different from the investigation of any feverish illness initially, but becomes more extensive if an early diagnosis is not forthcoming.

Caution.   Diagnosis is often much delayed and may be impossible after empirical treatment with antibiotics or corticosteroids. Although partial or transient improvement may be obtained, serological tests are altered and bacteriological cultures made impossible. While empirical treatment may be unavoidable if the patient is very ill, it should normally be deferred until most investigations have been completed or the diagnosis has been made.

The process of investigation falls conveniently into four stages which can usually be carried out in sequence at a pace which the patient can tolerate. If urgent investigation is indicated, components of the various stages can be carried out simultaneously.

Stage 1: immediate assessment
The various procedures of this stage are carried out on the day when the patient is first seen.

The clinical history.   This has two important functions; to ascertain the possibility of exposure to infection or allergen and to document the evolution of the illness.

The history of exposure should include contact with ill people, animals, farms, fresh water, also travel abroad, all medications both proprietary and prescribed and a family history of allergic or autoimmune conditions.

The evolution of the illness may suggest the diagnosis as it progresses and should therefore be recorded as accurately as possible.

Physical examination.   A lack of distinctive physical signs is usual in PUO, but subtle or doubtful signs may be all-important. Helpful signs include enlargement of lymph nodes, the appearance of nail haemorrhages, petechiae in the skin or mucous membranes, cytoid bodies or tubercles in the retina, pleural or pericardial friction rubs, persistent abdominal or renal tenderness, bone tenderness and cardiac murmurs.

The physical examination should be repeated daily for the first 2 or 3 days to check that minor abnormal physical signs are really present. After this initial period repeat examinations should be performed every few days or every week. This process makes easier the detection of slow changes in signs such as cardiac murmurs, enlargement of organs or gradual appearance of petechiae.

Tuberculin test.   If this is performed at the time of initial assessment it is unlikely to be omitted.

Immediate laboratory investigations.
   1. Chemical tests on urine: blood and protein can indicate urinary tract infection but are also seen in glomerulonephritis and neoplastic conditions.

Bile is present in prodromal hepatitis and infections of the biliary tree. It is also a sign of cholestasis.

Glucose usually indicates a diagnosis of diabetes mellitus which not uncommonly presents with a severe infection. Mild hyperglycaemia occurs in acute cerebral disorders and is usually transient.

2. Blood count and film: the white cell count can be a useful aid to diagnosis. In general, a high white cell count tends to be due to a neutrophil leukocytosis indicating probable bacterial infection, and a low count is due to neutropenia indicating probable viral infection. There are however important exceptions to this rule. Large increases in the white blood cell count can be due to lymphocytosis (common in whooping cough) or to eosinophilia (common in worm infestations). Neutropenia is seen in enteric fevers and brucellosis. A normal absolute count with over 90% polymorphs is seen in early staphylococcal septicaemia. A low count with normal differential is common in all types of overwhelming infection.

The red cells may contain parasites in malaria. They are slightly enlarged when haemolysis causes reticulocytosis, as in *Mycoplasma pneumoniae* infection.

3. The erythrocyte sedimentation rate (ESR): this can also be a very helpful immediate investigation. It is moderately raised, usually to no more than 50 mm per hour in many acute infections. A very high ESR of 80 mm per hour or more is seen in *Mycoplasma pneumoniae* infections, legionnaire's disease, drug reactions and collagen diseases.

4. The chest X-ray: this should be done early in all cases. Atypical pneumonias, tuberculosis, sarcoidosis, tumours and allergic pneumonitis can all produce gross X-ray changes in the absence of physical signs.

5. Bacteriology: blood, sputum, midstream urine, pus, faeces and, if indicated, cerebrospinal fluid should be obtained for microscopy and culture.

6. Virology: specimens as for bacteriology can be examined by electron microscopy and tissue culture techniques.

7. Obtain a reference serum sample: this will be available for various serological studies and in particular will provide the first serum for paired sera which are often used in the next stage.

Stage 2: serodiagnosis
This is the stage at which infections may be diagnosed by the detection of antibodies in the patient's serum. Some diagnoses can be made by examination of a single serum sample. These are usually disorders in which high titres of agglutinating antibodies appear early during illness or in which IgM antibodies are readily detectable. Some individual diseases produce unique antibody reactions which are also useful for rapid diagnosis. Most diagnoses, however, still rely on the finding of rising antibody titres in paired sera. A significant rise in titre cannot be expected in less than 2 weeks and sometimes takes longer than this to appear. In a

few cases a third or even fourth serum may be required in the third to sixth week of illness.

Stage 3: immunological disorders
This is the stage which is arrived at if stages 1 and 2 have failed to reveal an infectious disease, though it can be combined with stages 1 and 2 if autoimmune disease is strongly suspected. Earlier clinical and laboratory findings may guide the physician to suspect a particular disorder. In particular, arthritis, transient or fluctuating pleuritis or pneumonitis, and unusual rashes may arouse suspicion, especially if the ESR is high. Neutropenia is common in systemic lupus erythematosus and severe rheumatoid disease, while neutrophil leukocytosis is usually seen in polyarteritis nodosa and dermatomyositis.

In many autoimmune disorders the diagnosis rests on the finding of particular autoantibodies in the patient's serum. In sarcoidosis, a granulomatous disease, the Kveim test may be positive and the serum angiotensin-converting enzyme (SACE) is often elevated.

When serological testing is unhelpful or when the diagnosis requires confirmation, tissue diagnosis is necessary.

Stage 4: tissue diagnosis
This is the stage at which imaging and biopsy techniques are brought into play. There is no reason why these techniques cannot be employed during the first or second stages, as they may well be if early clinical and laboratory findings suggest that they are indicated. The best interpretation of images or of histology, however, often depends on the amount of background information available to the radiologist or pathologist. For this reason procedures which can be distressing to the patient are often carried out only when considerable information has already been accrued. Several techniques are available.

Ultrasound.   This is particularly useful for imaging of solid abdominal organs and of the female pelvis and it has the advantage of being noninvasive. It can demonstrate abscesses or cysts of the liver or kidneys, enlargement of the uterus and large abscesses of the peritoneal reflections. It can also reveal gallstones and dilatation of the biliary tree.

Echocardiography also employs ultrasonic emissions and can demonstrate vegetations on, or deformity of the heart valves, and pericardial effusions.

Biopsy techniques can be performed with the aid of ultrasonic imaging.

X-ray studies.   Both plain X-rays and contrast studies are useful. Sequences of chest or bone X-rays can show enlarging lesions. Cholecystography and contrast urography are widely used to demonstrate abnormalities of the biliary and renal tracts as well as parenchymal disorders of the kidneys.

Computerized scanning. This is particularly useful for the head, the spine and the solid abdominal viscera. Enlarged abdominal lymph nodes are often well-demonstrated.

Isotope scanning. This is useful particularly for visualizing the liver and the bones. Standard technetium scanning shows abscesses and defects due to cysts. Gallium scanning shows positive scintillation in areas of liver infiltrated by lymphoma.

Nuclear magnetic resonance imaging. This is a new technique which differs from the others in showing tissue metabolic activity. As tissue oedema is readily demonstrated, it may complement other scanning techniques in indicating sites of inflammation.

Needle biopsy techniques. These allow both culture and microscopic examination of tissues. Bone marrow, superficial lymph nodes, liver, kidney, pleura and superficial tumours are all relatively easy to sample by this technique. Skilled operators can needle lung tissue and abscesses of the liver and kidney.

Excision biopsy. This is preferred for enlarged lymph nodes and superficial tumours, as complete excision reduces the dissemination of any malignancy. Unfortunately inguinal lymph nodes often have bizarre histology and are therefore rarely welcomed by pathologists if axillary or cervical nodes are obtainable instead.

Laparoscopy. This is a relatively minor procedure which permits direct observation of abdominal and pelvic organs. It is particularly useful in the diagnosis of abdominopelvic tuberculosis and of disorders of abdominal lymph nodes. Lymph node biopsy can be performed at laparoscopy.

Diagnostic laparotomy. The development of high-resolution imaging techniques and of laparoscopy has probably much reduced the need for this major procedure. In some cases with persistent abdominal symptoms or where malignancy, particularly Hodgkin's disease which may be treatable, is suspected it still has an indispensable part to play.

Other operative investigations. Open bone biopsy is strongly recommended by many to confirm diagnosis and obtain material for culture in osteomyelitis, particularly as the evacuation of pus and sequestrum is often a major part of treatment.

Operative exploration of cerebral abscesses, subphrenic abscesses and other abdominal infections may also be mandatory.

Caution.   Negative results from imaging and biopsy techniques do not always exclude a diagnosis. The extent of the disease may be such that it is beyond the resolution of imaging techniques, or missed by the exploring needle. Subdural and subphrenic abscesses, pancreatic abscesses and cysts, and peritoneal infections are particularly difficult to demonstrate. If clinical signs contradict the evidence of images and biopsies, it may be as well to attend to the clinical signs.

The use of therapeutic trials

There is usually no place for therapeutic trial in the investigation of PUO. Apart from the fact that the treatment involved can prevent elucidation of the underlying problem, few patients with PUO will respond completely to empirical treatment. There are, however, a few exceptions to this principle.

Strong suspicion of autoimmune disease or hypersensitivity state

This situation arises when a patient has persistent, unchanging fever, raised ESR and often myalgia, fleeting rashes and evidence of liver dysfunction. Usually no diagnosis is evident after immunological investigations. It is important to perform liver biopsy which may show typical features of persisting infection, chronic hepatitis, drug-induced damage, granuloma or lymphoma, and to biopsy affected skin and muscle, which may show areas of chronic inflammation or vasculitis.

If other disorders are excluded and only non-specific chronic inflammatory changes are found, a trial of corticosteroids may be carried out, in case the patient has an ill-defined autoimmune condition.

All other medication, such as antihypertensive agents, should be discontinued or substituted so as to remove possible precipitating stimuli. Prednisolone 60–80 mg daily is then given, usually in divided doses.

The fever and raised ESR usually fall whatever the cause of illness, but if corticosteroid therapy is having beneficial effect the patient's sense of wellbeing will improve, his appetite return and abnormal liver function and other tests will return to normal. A response can usually be expected within a few days. After 7–10 days, dosage should either be 'tailed off' or gradually reduced to the minimum effective level.

Strong possibility of tuberculosis

A few feverish patients have a good history of exposure to tuberculosis or a strongly positive tuberculin test, but no confirmation of the infection is obtainable even by lymph node or liver biopsy. If no other cause of fever is found, a trial of antituberculous therapy is justified.

Unfortunately rifampicin and streptomycin are active against many bacteria, including pathogens capable of causing endocarditis. To avoid partial treatment of such conditions, only drugs whose effect is strictly

Table 14. Sequence of diagnostic procedures in PUO

	Stage 1: immediate	Stage 2: serological	Stage 3: immunological	Stage 4: tissue*
I	Septicaemias			
N	Meningitis			
F	Infectious mononucleosis			
E	Pneumonias			
C	Biliary infection			
T	Urinary infection			
I	Endocarditis			
O	Tuberculosis			
U	Abscesses			
S	Osteomyelitis			
		Single serum		
		Brucellosis		
		Syphilis		
		Toxoplasmosis		
		Amoebiasis		
		Paired sera		
		Viral infections		
I		*Mycoplasma*		
M		Q fever		
M		*Legionella*		
U		Rickettsiae		
N		Leptospira		
O		Chlamydiae		
L			Rheumatoid disease	
O			Sarcoidosis	
G			Systemic lupus erythematosus	
I			Chronic hepatitis	
C				Drug jaundice
A				Polyarteritis nodosa
L				Dermatomyositis
				Crohn's disease
N				Hodgkin's disease
E				Hypernephroma
O				Hepatoma
P				
L	Leukaemias			
A				Lymphomas
S				
T				
I				
C				

*Imaging and biopsy can confirm the diagnosis made in Stages 1, 2 and 3.

antituberculous should be used in therapeutic trials. A combination of ethambutol, pyrazinamide and isoniazid would be satisfactory (see Chapter 13), with the proviso that *Mycobacterium bovis* is resistant to pyrazinamide though rarely to the other two drugs.

Many patients with tuberculosis show some response to treatment within 1 week, but an unfortunate minority must take the drugs for several weeks before gradually improving. A trial of therapy should not be abandoned, therefore, until at least 6–8 weeks of treatment have been completed. If there is a response to therapy, rifampicin may be substituted for pyrazinamide to allow the benefits of shorter duration of treatment (again, see Chapter 13).

The patient's condition causes concern
Patients with persistent high fever are usually unable to eat and often sweat profusely. These factors combine with the catabolism resulting from fever and quickly produce a negative protein and electrolyte balance. Accompanying toxaemia or bacteraemia may make the prognosis very bleak. In this urgent situation there is no alternative but to embark on a vigorous programme of treatment in an effort to save life. The choice of treatment should be influenced by any clinical information so far available, but might be a combination of corticosteroids, antibiotics and intensive nutrition. Very wide-spectrum antibiotics are available, so complicated mixtures can usually be avoided. If the latest aminoglycosides, penicillins or cephalosporins are used, a narrow-spectrum penicillin and metronidazole may also be needed to account for Gram-positive cocci and Gram-negative anaerobes. In a difficult situation where a wide range of Gram-positive and Gram-negative organisms must be considered in conjunction with mycoplasmas, rickettsiae or *Legionella spp.* chloramphenicol can be a useful agent. Antituberculous agents can be added to the regimen if indicated.

Continuing efforts should be made to arrive at a diagnosis, as treatment can often then be simplified. Successful empirical treatment should be continued for a reasonable length of time, usually at least 2 weeks, to ensure eradication of infection. Antibiotics should then be discontinued. If all remains well, corticosteroids may then be 'tailed off' and antituberculous therapy stopped last of all. This sequential stopping of treatment may reveal which was the effective component if illness should recur.

19

Hospital Infection

Introduction
Infection is common in hospital populations. In Britain about 10% of hospital patients are admitted because of infection, and a similar number acquire infection after admission. Individual surveys suggest that the situation is similar in Europe and the United States of America.

Of those who are admitted to hospital with infection about 30% have lower respiratory infections, about 15% have urinary tract infections and only about 2% have infected wounds. Of those who become infected during admission only about 15% have respiratory infections, nearly 20% have wound infections and 30% have urinary tract infections. About 5% acquire bacteraemias.

Factors predisposing to hospital infection
Patients' susceptibilities. Patients with similar predispositions to infection tend to be grouped together in the same wards. This inescapable fact of hospital use affords an ideal environment for the perpetuation of some infections (Table 15).

Possible foci of infection in hospitals

Infected patients
The infected patient often contaminates his immediate surroundings with pathogens. The most densely contaminated areas include the pillow and lower sheet of the bed, the patient's bedclothes, urinals, urine drainage bags, bedpans and dressings. Any nurse, medical attendant, domestic worker, visitor or other patient who handles these articles is likely to acquire pathogens on the hands, and may transfer sufficient numbers to themselves or another individual to cause a new infection. Fortunately most of these people remember to wash their hands between attending to different patients. Ordinary hand-washing with any soap is extremely effective in removing contamination.

Few serious illnesses spread by the airborne route in hospital. Notable exceptions are the childhood infectious diseases, influenza and pulmonary tuberculosis. Even when patients with these diseases are isolated in single rooms, airborne organisms may exit via ventilation systems or on air currents through doorways and other openings. Strict control of such infections therefore demands special isolation facilities.

Table 15.   Some predispositions to hospital-acquired infection

Ward	Type of predisposition	Resulting infection
Medical	Diabetic ulcer	
	trophic	Gram-positive infections
	ischaemic	Gram-negative and anaerobic infections
	Glycosuria	Urinary tract infections
Surgical	Skin incisions	Gram-positive infections
	Bowel surgery	Gram-negative skin infections Abdominal abscesses
Urological	Bladder catheters	Urinary tract infections
	Cytoscopy/instrumentation	Gram-negative bacteraemia
	Prostatic biopsy	
Geriatric	Incontinence	Urinary tract infections
	Pressure sores	Mixed Gram-negative infections
Intensive care	Endotracheal tubes	Hypostatic chest infections
	Bladder catheters	Urinary tract infections
	Intravenous cannulae	Cellulitis and bacteraemia
	Wide-spectrum antibiotics	Infections with very resistant organisms
Oncology	Immune suppression	Opportunistic infections
Many	Regular antibiotic use	Infections with resistant organisms

The hospital fixtures and fittings
Worktops.   Dusty worktops (and floors) can harbour staphylococci, streptococci, fungi and spores. Such contamination is easily removed by vacuum cleaning and damp dusting.

Damp surfaces and equipment.   Surfaces which are permanently damp can harbour Gram-negative bacteria, including *Klebsiella*, *Serratia* and *Pseudomonas*, which survive well in stagnant water and sometimes even in unused disinfectant solutions. Damp mops and cloths are ideal habitats for such organisms. Precautions against such contamination include the drying of damp-dusted or wetted surfaces, emptying and draining buckets, hanging up mops and cloths to dry and discarding unused disinfectant solutions.

Sinks and baths.   These can suffer from two major contamination problems. The first is persisting damp or wet areas. Some of this is due to ill-maintained, dripping taps and some to permanent wet areas such as water traps (U-bends). Water traps are usually cleansed by frequent rapid flow of water through them, but if they become blocked or stagnant they then present a hazard.

The other main problem, also concerned with maintenance, is the presence of cracks which provide a lodgement for organisms and cannot be adequately cleaned. Staphylococcal and streptococcal infection has been spread among successive patients using the same chipped bath.

The potential problem of contamination of taps by people wishing to wash their hands is overcome by the provision of elbow- or foot-operated taps.

If the equipment is well-maintained, cleaning with mild scouring agents and detergent will remove pathogens adequately.

Hospital equipment. The safety of equipment such as anaesthetic machines, cystoscopes, gastroscopes and respiratory function testing equipment is a serious problem. Outbreaks of tuberculosis and salmonellosis have resulted from faulty disinfection of such instruments. All-metal items can be sterilized by heating, but rubber articles and fibroptic equipment cannot. The use of chemical disinfectants is of value in some cases but precleaning by hand must be done to remove organic matter, which inactivates disinfectants.

The use of disposable microfilters, airways and tubing for ventilators has solved some cleansing problems.

The various methods of controlling infection

Surveillance and investigation
This enables the early detection and eradication of infections in a hospital. Since most episodes of infection come to the notice of the microbiology department in the normal course of diagnosis, this is the usual starting-point of surveillance. A *Control of Infection Officer* often takes part. He collates all information on episodes of infection, and notes any existing or emerging problems. It is convenient if this officer is a *Control of Infection Nursing Officer*, who understands nursing procedures and can cooperate with ward staff in finding the source and means of transmission of the infection.

In a large hospital the Control of Infection Nursing Officer can often discuss the matter with a *Control of Infection Committee* which may include microbiologists, physicians, surgeons, domestic supervisors, sterile supplies officer, engineers and hospital administrators. Such a committee is able to recommend alterations in hospital procedures, or special action to terminate the spread of infection and to prevent further episodes.

Isolation of infected patients
This physically removes the risk of direct, patient-to-patient spread of infection. It does not, however, eliminate the risk of infection to nursing and other attendants, nor the risk that such attendants will carry the infection to other patients. The responsibility for infection control in these circumstances falls largely on nursing staff, but doctors, domestics,

medical students, physiotherapists and others should remember that they are not exempt from ward procedures.

The single most effective control of infection measure is to wash the hands after handling the patient or any article in his room. Close-woven gowns or coverall aprons are useful in preventing direct contamination of attendants' clothing, but it is very doubtful whether face masks afford protection against airborne infection and few units now use them. The use of latex or plastic gloves is controversial; they certainly offer no advantage over hand-washing alone, but there are strong medicolegal pressures for their use in handling hepatitis B antigen positive blood and certain other materials. (Gloves do not prevent inoculation accidents, they are just as easily perforated as is skin). A situation in which it is definitely of benefit to wear gloves is that in which the wearer has a skin lesion, such as a cut, abrasion or eczematous area. Gloves will prevent contamination of the broken skin.

The patient's room and its equipment should be kept scrupulously clean and dusted, to prevent establishment of the organism in the environment.

Disinfection and sterilization
Disinfection is the removal or destruction of some contaminating micro-organisms from an item. The term does not imply that the item is completely free of organisms, only that contamination has been reduced to an acceptable level for the item's intended use. A proctoscope, for instance, does not need to be as free of contamination as an intravenous cannula or an artificial heart valve.

Sterilization is the removal of all microbial contaminants, including spores which are resistant to boiling and to most chemicals.

Disinfection by cleaning. This is the most economical and effective means of reducing contamination of the environment. Soaps and detergents make the removal of dirt and grease very easy and they have some bacteriocidal effects of their own. Cleaning cloths and mops can be laundered and dried regularly, or disposables can be used.

Chemical disinfectants. These have several hidden disadvantages. They are only effective against certain organisms and can play a part in 'selecting' a resistant environmental flora. Some Gram-negative bacteria and certain yeasts can survive in diluted disinfectant solutions, and this fact shortens the usable shelf-life of many compounds. Disinfectants must not be kept long enough to develop microbial contamination.

All chemical disinfectants are inactivated by organic matter. They cannot, therefore, be used effectively in soiled areas or on unwashed equipment.

Most disinfectants are liable to cause skin irritation in people who come into regular contact with them. This limits the usefulness of some agents, such as glutaraldehyde.

Disinfection by heat.   There are three ways of decontaminating articles by the use of heat.

1. *Pasteurization* is the use of heat to kill vegetative organisms. Heating to 80 °C will kill most bacteria and fungi. It will not destroy spores, which can germinate after pasteurization if they encounter favourable conditions. Pasteurization is used to clean many articles when contamination by some spores is acceptable. Bedpan-washers and laundry washing machines operate at 80 °C or above. Boiling pasteurizers are used to disinfect scissors, aural specula, proctoscopes, contaminated receptacles and crockery.

2. *Wet heat (steam sterilization)* is the most widely applied method of removing all microbial contamination, including spores. The *autoclave* is the machine in which steam under pressure is used to reach the necessary high temperatures for complete sterilization. The pressures and temperatures can be tested either by direct measurement, or by the addition of Brownes tubes to the load in the autoclave. The Brownes tubes contain liquids which change colour under certain well-defined temperature conditions, and provide a rapid test of autoclave function.

Gamma rays.   High doses of gamma rays can kill all organisms including spores. Many organic compounds such as paper, plastic and latex are transparent to gamma rays and are readily sterilized by them. Items such as disposable syringes, catheters and cannulae are presealed into airtight containers and then sterilized by gamma irradiation. The interior of the package remains sterile until the seal is broken.

Production of intense gamma irradiation is expensive and requires extensive plant. This method of sterilization is therefore more applicable to industrial production than to hospital use.

Opportunistic infections

Introduction
An opportunistic infection is one which would not be expected to occur in a patient with normal body defences (Table 16). Such infections may be unusual for any of several reasons.

The patient might have expected to be immune.   This is the case when previously immune patients who have a defect of cell-mediated immunity develop new or reactivated tuberculosis. The classical situation is that in which a patient with known lymphoma develops new lymph-node swelling due to tuberculous granuloma, or suffers from destructive pulmonary disease.

Table 16.   Some examples of opportunistic infections

Condition	Predisposing factors	Common infections
Endotracheal intubation, mucoviscidosis, dust diseases	Defective clearance pathogens from bronchial tree	Chest infections including staphylococcal and Gram-negative infections
Rheumatic heart disease, heart valve implants, CSF shunts	Tissue or implant inaccessible to immune reaction	Serious infections following trivial bacteraemias; organisms of low pathogenicity, e.g. *Staph. epidermidis* or diphtheroids
Agammaglobulinaemia	Deficient humoral immunity	Bacterial infections, particularly respiratory and urinary infection
Lymphomas and lymphocytic leukaemias	Deficient cell-mediated immunity	Tuberculosis Severe chickenpox and other viral infections Cryptococcal meningitis
Splenectomy	Defective clearance of bacteria from bloodstream	Pneumococcal and other bacteraemias
Transplant patients	Immunosuppressive drugs (mainly against cell-mediated response)	Viral and fungal infections, cytomegalovirus pneumonitis, tuberculosis
Treated leukaemias, bone marrow transplants	Multiple cytotoxic agents; background of abnormal immune reactions	Bacteraemias and septicaemias, cytomegalovirus pneumonitis and viraemia, *Pneumocystis carinii* pneumonitis
Some groups of homosexual men, intravenous drug abusers and their contacts	Deficient cell-mediated immunity (acquired immuno-deficiency syndrome or AIDS)	Life threatening herpes simplex and cytomegalovirus infections, aggressive Kaposi's sarcoma, *Pneumocystis carinii* pneumonia

The clinical course of an infection is unusual.   Many of the clinical features of infections are partly caused by the patient's immune reactions, and the eventual resolution of the disease is also dependent on the immune response. In opportunistic infections the course of the disease may be abnormal: in deficiencies of cell-mediated responses granulomas may fail to form, or chickenpox and herpes simplex lesions may fail to heal; in granulocyte deficiencies pus may fail to form, there may be no inflammatory exudate and the features of endotoxaemia may be modified; infection is not necessarily accompanied by fever. In many cases localizing signs are not seen, partly because infection quickly becomes disseminated and partly because of failure of local responses. A good example of this is the chest X-ray in opportunistic lung infections, in which the disease may be so diffuse that no radiographic lesion is demonstrable, or at best a vague ground-glass or diffuse nodular appearance is seen.

The infecting organism is not usually a pathogen. This is a common circumstance, seen when an organism which is usually a harmless part of the normal body flora overcomes weakened body defences and causes infection. Severe infections with *Staphylococcus epidermidis* or *Candida albicans* from the skin, *Strep. viridans* or faecal streptococci from the mouth or the genital tract, and Gram-negative organisms such as *Pseudomonas spp.*, *Serratia spp.*, *Citrobacter* and *Acinetobacter* are all commonly opportunistic. Less common, but also significant hazards are *Cryptococcus*, *Aspergillus* and *Nocardia* infections.

Caution. Immunocompromised patients are just as easily attacked by recognized pathogens as by unusual ones. It is a mistake to forget this.

Recognition of opportunistic infection
This depends on an understanding of the patient's predisposition to such infections and the vigilance of the physician for subtle alterations in the patient's condition. Many develop fever and an alteration in blood count during episodes of infection, but some are unable to produce such responses because of immune deficiency. Signs such as tachycardia, breathing difficulties, cough and sputum should be taken seriously even in the absence of fever.

Laboratory investigations. The diagnosis of opportunistic infection is usually an urgent matter, and vigorous investigation is carried out at an early stage. This may include blood, urine and sputum cultures, search for serological evidence of fungal and viral infections, bronchoscopy and even lung biopsy if *Pneumocystis carinii* is suspected. Laboratory results of 'doubtful significance', such as a finding of micrococci or diphtheroids in blood cultures, should be treated seriously because such organisms may be pathogens in an immunodeficient patient.

Treatment of opportunistic infections
In most cases it is unacceptable to delay treatment while awaiting the diagnosis. As soon as satisfactory cultural and serological samples are obtained, 'blunderbuss' therapy is commenced. There is some opportunity for intelligent guesswork to guide therapy if the site or nature of infection is known; in particular *Pneumocystis carinii* is a fairly common chest pathogen in leukaemics on cytotoxic therapy, but the range of potential pathogens is very wide and the spectrum of treatment must be correspondingly broad. It is usual to give, intravenously, a combination of bacteriocidal agents such as benzylpenicillin, a wide-spectrum

cephalosporin or aminoglycoside and metronidazole. Co-trimoxazole in approximately twice the normal dosage is often useful in treating *Pneumocystis* infections. The search for antiviral agents active against cytomegalovirus has not yet been successful, but herpes simplex and varicella zoster will often respond to antiviral agents.

Treatment is continued according to the patient's response and any information available after microbiological investigation.

In some cases immunoglobulin, such as human normal immunoglobulin may improve deficient humoral immunity, granulocyte transfusion may assist the response to bacterial infection and plasmapheresis may remove toxins from the bloodstream.

Prevention of opportunistic infection
Segregation of susceptibles from sources of infection.   This requires considerable planning and administration. It means strict observation of hospital hygiene and cleaning procedures, exclusion of workers with even trivial infections from oncology and transplant units, assurance that staff do not pass directly from infected areas to the oncology unit, and avoidance of infecting susceptible patients with live vaccines. Attention to this type of detail will prevent patients becoming cross-infected while in hospital, but cannot prevent them from being infected by normal body flora or environmental organisms.

Prophylactic medication.   This has had little success in the past, except in the prevention of rheumatic fever and of bacterial endocarditis, when it is thought by most to be essential.

Prophylaxis against rheumatic fever is successful because treatment is aimed at only one organism, *Streptococcus pyogenes*, which does not become resistant to the appropriate antibiotic, benzylpenicillin. This situation is rare, as many organisms in the normal body flora are able to become resistant to antibiotics of various types. In addition to this, removal of sensitive flora leaves areas of the body available for colonization by more resistant organisms. Any prophylactic medication, therefore, loses its usefulness as soon as the sensitive flora have been replaced, usually in a few days.

Short-term prophylaxis can be useful if the time when the patient will be in danger is predictable. Thus sudden, brief bacteraemias during dental treatment, bladder instrumentation, prostatic biopsy, endoscopic retrograde cholecystopancreatography and surgical procedures, can be forestalled by short courses of antibiotics. It is usual to give the antibiotics so that the peak blood level coincides with the anticipated bacteraemia. Further doses may be given over approximately 2 more days whilst surgical incisions and biopsy wounds stabilize.

Middle-term prophylaxis is used for leukaemic and other oncology patients during intensive cytotoxic treatment. It is impossible to eradicate all of the normal flora, which may invade the defenceless patient, but the load of organisms can be much reduced. The major load is in the bowel, and this is attacked with a mixture of non-absorbable antibiotics such as framycetin, colistin and nystatin. The skin is washed with disinfectant solutions and creams are applied to the external nares and the perineum. Organisms will remain in the dental clefts, and recesses of the bowel and genital tracts, but their numbers are relatively few. Strict isolation in filtered-air rooms or plastic envelopes is sometimes employed to prevent recolonization by environmental organisms. Few patients can tolerate such regimens for very long because of distressing diarrhoea and the local effects of disinfectant applications, but many specialists feel that the reduced risk of infection permits more effective cytotoxic therapy.

Long-term chemoprophylaxis against infection is rarely used. An exception to this rule is co-trimoxazole prophylaxis against *Pneumocystis carinii* infection in patients on prolonged cytotoxic therapy. This is thought to offer a very significant level of protection and is of considerable benefit. Other forms of long-term prophylaxis, such as tetracycline prophylaxis for bronchitis, low-dose trimethoprim or co-trimoxazole for recurrent urinary infections, and co-trimoxazole for chest infections in patients with mucoviscidosis, are more controversial. Some physicians feel that repeated short courses of treatment offer similar benefits without encouraging the development of a resistant body flora.

Immunization.   Immunization against surface antigens of *Pseudomonas* has been carried out experimentally, and appears to protect patients with extensive burns from *Pseudomonas* bacteraemia.

Immunization against endotoxin may give some protection against Gram-negative bacteraemias.

20

Immunization

Introduction
Immunization is the process of induction of immunity. Ancient Asian and African people are known to have procured immunity against smallpox by skin inoculation of lymph from the lesions of mild cases (variolation). This was often effective, but the risk of fatal disease, and indeed of an epidemic, was considerable. In 1796 Jenner demonstrated that inoculation of lymph from cowpox lesions (vaccination) would produce immunity against smallpox, and the word *vaccine* is now applied to all antigenic agents which are used to stimulate an immune response.

Active immunization
This term is applied when immunity is induced by antigens. The antigens may be (a) avirulent versions of the wild pathogen (*live vaccines*), (b) killed pathogens or extracts of pathogens, or (c) altered bacterial toxins, called toxoids. Killed pathogens and toxoids are constituents of *inactivated vaccines*.

Passive immunization
The role of antibodies in immune responses was discovered at the end of last century, though the use of antisera in the treatment of disease has become relatively rare since antibiotics have been so successful. It is possible, however, to confer temporary immunity by giving parenteral doses of antisera. Since the antisera are mainly proteins, they are gradually metabolized by the recipient and lose their effect in 3–6 months.

Thus passive immunization provides a degree of protection as soon as it is given, in contrast to active immunization whose effect is delayed until the recipient's immune system has responded sufficiently. It has the disadvantage of being very short-lasting compared with active immunization which, at its best, can last more or less indefinitely.

Live Vaccines

These vaccines contain live organisms of attenuated pathogenicity (Table 17). Each batch of vaccine is prepared by direct subculture from the pool of original organisms, so that repeated subculturing cannot pro-

Table 17. Examples of live vaccines

Name	Cultured in
BCG (Bacillus Calmette–Guérin)	Chemical media
Measles vaccine	Chick embryo cells
Mumps vaccine	Chick embryo cells
Oral polio vaccine (Sabin)	Monkey kidney cells
Rubella vaccine	Rabbit kidney, duck embryo or human cells
Yellow fever vaccine	Chick embryos

duce successive generations of organisms with increasing pathogenicity.

The vaccine viruses are often raised in animal tissue cultures. Antibiotics are added to the cultures to prevent bacterial contamination. The tissues and antibiotics may vary depending on the type of vaccine and the manufacturer.

The storage of live vaccines can be a problem as the organisms are killed by deep-freezing as well as by warming. Freeze-drying makes shelf-storage easy. Otherwise the vaccines must be stored at 4 °C. Once reconstituted, diluted or opened the vaccine must be promptly used, and any excess discarded.

Effects of live vaccines
Immunity is induced by causing a mild or subclinical infection. Vaccine viruses can often be recovered from the pharynx or the faeces of the recipient for a time after immunization. As vaccine viruses cause viraemia, just as virulent viruses do, they may be dangerous in certain circumstances.

In pregnancy. The fetus has an immature immune response and could possibly suffer severe infection even with an attenuated virus. Live vaccines should not therefore be given to pregnant women, though no ill-effects from accidental administration during pregnancy have been reported so far. Even so, termination of pregnancy may be considered if a woman accidentally receives rubella vaccine in the first trimester or in the 12 weeks preceding conception. (Oral polio vaccine may be given after the fourth month of pregnancy, or earlier in an emergency).

In immune deficiency. The unopposed attenuated pathogen can produce severe opportunistic infection. In the case of oral polio vaccine, prolonged faecal excretion occurs, and carries the danger of the virus reverting to a virulent form.

Live vaccines also have important advantages. Their natural stimulation of immunity means that a single dose is usually all that is required to procure an adequate immune response. (Three doses of oral polio vaccine are given, as it contains three different strains of virus). In addition to this, attenuated viruses can compete with live viruses. Oral polio virus, for instance, given during a polio epidemic, can colonize the bowel mucosa and deny access to the wild virus. It has also been given to neonates in an attempt to interfere with epidemics of ECHOvirus infection.

Adverse effects of live vaccines
Mild infection. This is the most common effect, and takes the form of a mild fever, sometimes with a rash, after an incubation period. The patient rarely feels ill.

Allergic reactions. Local skin reactions sometimes occur, caused by antigens of the vaccine organism or foreign proteins from the tissue culture. They are usually trivial.

Generalized reactions occur rarely, and are minimized if the patient is asked about allergy to animals, animal proteins and antibiotics *before* immunization. If there is a history of allergy, the constituents of the vaccine should be ascertained in case it cannot safely be given.

Reversion of vaccine organisms to virulence. This is exceedingly rare, but is known to occur in about one per million oral polio immunizations. Either the recipient or his unvaccinated contacts may then develop paralytic disease. For this reason unimmunized parents should receive the vaccine at the same time as their child's primary course.

Inactivated polio vaccine is as effective as the live vaccine in conferring immunity, and is the preferred agent in some countries.

Interference with the effect of other live vaccines. If more than one live vaccine must be given, dosage should either be simultaneous or the vaccines should be given at least 3 weeks apart.

Inactivated vaccines

Some of the organisms used in the vaccines are heat-killed. Others, and the toxoids, are inactivated by a reaction with formalin. Inactivated vaccines may contain traces of formalin, foreign protein derived from culture media, and preservatives such as phenol.

Adsorbed vaccines. Inactivated vaccines can be made more antigenic by the addition of certain substances called adjuvants. Pertussis vaccine itself has an adjuvant effect on the other components of triple vaccine.

Most of the inactivated vaccines for use in childhood are available as preparations adsorbed onto aluminium salts. These preparations are pre-

Table 18.   Examples of inactivated vaccines

Killed organisms or antigenic extracts	Toxoids
Cholera vaccine	Diphtheria toxoid
Hepatitis B vaccine	Tetanus toxoid
Group A and C meningococcal vaccines	
Pertussis vaccine	
Pneumococcal vaccine	
Polio vaccine	
(Salk vaccine)	
Typhoid vaccine	
Human diploid cell rabies vaccine	
Vaccines against anthrax, plague, typhus and Weil's disease	

ferred to plain vaccines both for their enhanced antigenicity and because of their low propensity for causing systemic reactions. Local reactions, however, are more common after adsorbed than after plain vaccines, and adsorbed vaccines must not be given intradermally as they produce persisting skin nodules.

Effects of inactivated vaccines
As they only present a brief antigenic stimulus instead of a true infection, these vaccines do not stimulate effective immunity after a single dose. The first dose produces a small, transient, rise in IgM antibody levels, the *primary response*, which indicates that the immune system has learned to recognize the antigen. If a further dose is given immediately it will provoke no more reaction. A second dose after an interval of a few weeks, however, produces a sudden large rise in IgG antibody levels, which is sustained. This is the *secondary response* which provides immunity. A third dose of vaccine after a longer interval may produce a still higher sustained antibody level, which can be maintained by occasional reinforcing doses.

Adverse effects
Hypersensitivity reactions.   These are often caused by the protein components of the vaccine, or the antigens themselves. Anaphylaxis is extremely rare and often follows a second dose when there has been a lesser reaction to the first.

   Subcutaneous nodules may appear after injection of adsorbed vaccines. They are painless and harmless, eventually resolving spontaneously.

Idiosyncratic reactions.   These also are extremely rare in their severe forms. Restlessness, mild fever and screaming attacks are well-recognized mild reactions to triple vaccine (diphtheria/tetanus/pertussis) and are usually ascribed to the pertussis component, though they can also occur after measles immunization.

The more serious reactions including convulsions, encephalopathy and cerebral damage are thought to occur in not more than one in 100 000 to 300 000 immunizations. The majority of severe reactions are, again, thought due to pertussis vaccine and the risk is mainly confined to those who have a history of cerebral irritability or disorder.

Contraindications to pertussis immunization
Absolute
1. severe local, neurological or general reaction to a previous dose.
2. a history of cerebral irritation, neonatal cerebral injury, fits or convulsions.

Strong
1. parents or siblings have a history of epilepsy.
2. developmental delay is present which is thought to be due to a neurological defect.
3. there is existing neurological disease.
(these contraindications might also be reasons for considering pertussis immunization during epidemic years, but only if they occur when the infant is in the high-risk group of those below age 3 years)

Other vaccines have been recognized as causing rare cases of encephalitis. Rabies vaccines derived from animal brain tissue and smallpox vaccine were among the most common offenders, but there is now little need to use them as in the first case human diploid cell vaccine is safer and better, and in the second case the need for immunization has been eradicated.

Passive immunization

Effects of antisera
Antisera (Table 19) are usually given by intramuscular injection. In severe diphtheria or botulism part of the dose may be given intravenously, and in rabies prophylaxis it is usual to give half of the dose by infiltration into the injured tissues.

These means of administration provide immediately detectable antibody levels. In prophylaxis the aim of this is to neutralize circulating viruses or bacterial toxins before they can become fixed in the tissues. Early use is therefore essential, and a prophylactic effect cannot usually be guaranteed if prophylaxis is delayed for more than 2 days after exposure.

When used in treatment antisera are rarely thought to be curative, but are given in an attempt to neutralize bloodborne viruses or toxins and therefore prevent further tissue damage. They may be combined with other treatments, as in diphtheria.

Table 19. Examples of antisera

		Use
Human sera		
Human normal immunoglobulin	HNIG	Hepatitis A, measles, rubella (prophylaxis)
Hepatitis B immune globulin	HBIG	Hepatitis B prophylaxis
Human tetanus immune globulin	HTIG	Tetanus prophylaxis
Human rabies immune globulin	HRIG	Rabies prophylaxis
Zoster immune globulin	ZIG	Chickenpox prophylaxis (treatment in immune suppressed)
(Vaccinia immune globulin)	VIG	Treatment of systemic infection with smallpox vaccine virus
Mumps immune globulin		Prevention of mumps in immune-suppressed
Horse sera		
Diphtheria antitoxin		Diphtheria treatment
Botulinum antitoxin (monovalent and polyvalent)		Botulism treatment and prophylaxis

A further use of antisera is to provide temporary protection whilst active immunization takes effect, as in rabies and tetanus prophylaxis.

Adverse effects
Hypersensitivity reactions. These are rare when human immunoglobulins are used, but are a real risk when equine preparations must be given. When using animal sera a small test dose should usually be given, with adrenaline, antihistamines and corticosteroids at hand in case anaphylaxis should occur. If there is no adverse reaction the main dose is given after half an hour. In a crisis the test dose may have to be omitted.

Serum sickness is a delayed reaction which occurs several hours after treatment in a patient who is previously sensitized to the serum. It is a feverish illness with myalgia, arthralgia, sometimes a vasculitic rash and occasionally bronchoconstriction. Symptoms usually resolve spontaneously.

Inactivation of live vaccines. Some antisera can produce antibody levels capable of destroying attenuated organisms. Measles vaccine is inactivated in this way if given within 3 months of HNIG.

Applications of immunization

It may not be obvious on first consideration that the various effects of immunization allow its use for several different purposes.

Protection of the immunized individual

This is an obvious purpose of immunization and indeed, whatever other reasons there may be for immunizing an individual, personal protection will result. Some immunizations are strictly for individual protection, as are tetanus and rabies immunization, for these diseases are contracted by unique individual contact and do not pass from man to man. Others, like pertussis immunization, do not afford complete individual protection, but do have an overall effect in the community.

To increase herd immunity

An epidemic pathogen relies on a significant pool of susceptible individuals in its host population in order to continue its lifecycle. If the proportion of susceptibles falls below a certain level the progress of the pathogen through the population is inhibited. Even if not every host is immunized and if those immunized are not completely protected, sufficient fall in the transmission of a pathogen can be achieved. In this way the size of pertussis epidemics had been gradually reduced in Britain since immunization became available, until a fall in the acceptance of immunization was suddenly followed by epidemics as large as those seen 20 years previously (Fig. 26).

To protect another individual

Rubella immunization is a good example of this. Girls are not immunized to protect themselves, for rubella is almost always a trivial disease; they

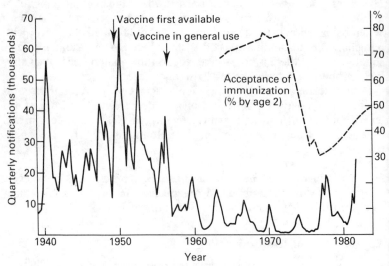

Fig. 26. Effect of immunization on pertussis epidemics in England and Wales (CDSC).

are immunized so that they cannot later transmit the disease to their developing fetus if they are exposed to rubella during pregnancy.

Immunization with inactivated vaccines may be performed during pregnancy with benefit to the fetus. If a woman receives tetanus toxoid and reaches a peak of immunity at the end of pregnancy, her baby is protected from neonatal tetanus, an important asset in some parts of the world.

To inhibit the progress of epidemics

This is a relatively limited application, but it can be used to great effect. Smallpox outbreaks were confined and eventually eradicated in this way. All immediate family, work and leisure contacts of a case are immunized as soon as possible. When this is achieved the secondary contacts (contacts of primary contacts and users of the same buildings, restaurants etc as the initial case) are immunized. If a contact develops the disease, *his* secondary contacts are promptly immunized. this is called the *expanding ring technique*. It works best when the disease is transmitted from person to person, for a vector might bypass the 'ring'. Oral polio vaccine can be used in this way, permitting greater economy of personnel and materials than a 'mass immunization' campaign. A live-attenuated chickenpox vaccine may soon be available, and could be used in this way.

The immunization programme in the United Kingdom

These immunizations are offered (but are not compulsory) to all eligible individuals free of charge. Other immunizations are available, but a small charge is usually made for them.

During the first year of life

Triple vaccine (diphtheria toxoid, tetanus toxoid and pertussis vaccine, adsorbed, or DTPer/Vac/Ads). This is given in three consecutive doses, the first two doses separated by 6–8 weeks and the second and third dose by 4–6 months.

The first dose should be given at 3 months of age. This is a compromise between obtaining an adequate response from the immature immune system and providing early protection against pertussis.

Diphtheria and tetanus toxoids (DT/Vac/Ads). This vaccine is used if there is a contraindication to the pertussis component of triple vaccine.

Oral polio vaccine (OPV or Pol/Vac (Oral)). This is given at the same times as the three doses of triple vaccine. Breast feeding does not inactivate Pol/Vac (Oral), but it is reasonable to avoid giving the vaccine together with a feed.

Unimmunized parents should receive Pol/Vac (Oral) when their child is immunized (see above).

During the second year of life
Measles vaccine (Meas/Vac (Live)).   This cannot be given before the age of 1 year, as it may be inactivated by long-lasting maternal antibodies. It is usually offered at 13 months.

At entry to nursery or infants' school

DT/Vac/Ads and Pol/Vac (Oral).   These should preferably be given at least 3 years after completion of the basic course.

Girls aged 10–14 years

Rubella vaccine (Rub/Vac (Live)).   This is given regardless of a history of rubella, which may well be unreliable.
   This vaccine may also be offered to susceptible adult women provided that they are warned to avoid pregnancy for 3 months after immunization.

At age 11–13 years

Immunization against tuberculosis (Tub/Vac/BCG).   This is offered to tuberculin-negative individuals. It may also be given to neonates who are likely to be tuberculosis contacts and to tuberculin-negative contacts of any age.
   Great care must be taken to give this preparation *intracutaneously*. Subcutaneous or intramuscular administration will cause a persistent 'cold abscess'.

On leaving school
Tet/Vac/Ads.

Pol/Vac (Oral).

In adulthood
Primary tetanus immunization (Tet/Vac/Ads).   This may be offered at any age, and may be begun when human tetanus immunoglobulin is offered for post-exposure prophylaxis.

Pol/Vac (Oral).   Booster doses are recommended before travel abroad to endemic areas.

Pol/Vac (Inact) (Salk vaccine).   This is an alternative to Pol/Vac (Oral). It is useful when the oral vaccine is contraindicated, as in pregnancy. In some countries it is preferred to the oral vaccine as it is equally effective and does not carry any risk of virulence.

Rabies vaccine. Human diploid cell-inactivated rabies vaccine, together with human rabies immunoglobulin, is offered to any individual who has been exposed to rabies.

Immunization schedules in other countries.

Republic of Ireland
Here, BCG is offered to neonates.

United States of America
Triple vaccine and oral polio vaccine are given at 2, 4 and 6 months of age. Boosters are given at age 18 months. BCG is not offered routinely.

Canada, United States and some European countries
Mumps immunization is offered routinely. It is available as a measles/rubella/mumps (live) combination offered at 12–15 months of age.

21

Postinfectious Disorders

Introduction
Not every patient regains normal health immediately after recovering
from an acute infection. Some develop new inflammatory lesions and
abnormal physical signs which are distinct from the original illness.

A number of postinfectious conditions are recognized (Table 20). Most
of them have features similar to inflammatory or autoimmune diseases,

Table 20. Known and suspected postinfectious disorders

Disorder	Associated infections
Multisystem diseases	
Rheumatic fever	*Strep. pyogenes* tonsillitis
Reiter's syndrome	Non-specific urethritis
	Bacillary dysentery
? Henoch–Schönlein syndrome	Streptococcal infections
	Upper respiratory infections
? Reye's syndrome	Chickenpox, mild respiratory infections
	Influenza B
	Drugs and toxins may be involved
? Lupus syndrome	Infectious mononucleosis
Arthropathies	
Large-joint or sacroiliitis	Meningococcal disease
	Bowel infections, especially *Yersinia* and *Klebsiella*
	Mumps (rare)
Small-joint	Rubella, other viral infections
Glomerulonephritis	*Strep. pyogenes* throat and skin diseases
	Staphylococcal infection (rare)
	Atypical pneumonias
	Viral infections (rare)
	Chronic malaria
Cardiac disorders	
Pericarditis	Coxsackie and other viral infections
	Meningococcal disease
Myocarditis	Coxsackie and other viral infections
Nervous system disease	
Encephalitis	Mumps, measles, chickenpox and other viral infections

Disorder	Associated infections
Neuropathies (including Guillain–Barré syndrome)	Infectious mononucleosis, cytomegalovirus infection, influenza and mild respiratory infections
Skin eruptions	
Erythema multiforme	Streptococcal infections
	Herpes simplex and other viral infections
	Antibiotics and other drugs
Erythema nodosum	Primary tuberculosis
	Yersinia and other bowel infections
	Leprosy
? 'Aesthenic' syndromes	Viral hepatitis
	Infectious mononucleosis
	Coxsackie group B and other viral infections
	Trivial 'viral' infections
Acquired immunodeficiency syndrome (AIDS)	?Parenterally transmitted infection
? Human tumours	Hepatoma in HBeAg-positive individuals
	Lymphomas following Epstein–Barr virus infections
	Carcinoma of the cervix following herpes simplex type II infections

with synovitis, vasculitis and glomerulonephritis among the commonest manifestations. Such disorders tend to appear within 2–3 weeks of an acute infection and usually resolve spontaneously after a variable period of time. A few, like rheumatic fever, can recur after repeated infections and eventually cause permanent tissue damage.

Recognition of postinfectious disorders can be important. Some, like Stevens–Johnson syndrome, can be ameliorated by early treatment. The effect of others, like rheumatic fever, can be minimized by preventing recurrent episodes. In a few cases the postinfectious disorder can reveal a previously unrecognized infection.

Pathogenesis of postinfectious disorders
There are several alternative hypotheses for the development of these disorders. Several factors probably combine to produce a wide spectrum of disease. A variety of conditions, for instance can follow *Streptococcus pyogenes* infection, including rheumatic fever, nephritis and vasculitic rashes; different mechanisms are probably responsible for each condition.

The susceptibility of the patient. In some cases it is possible to recognize features which indicate susceptibility to particular postinfectious disorders. Patients who do not secrete blood-group substances in their body fluids (non-secretors) are known to be more susceptible to rheumatic fever than are secretors. Patients with tissue type HLA B27 are susceptible to Reiter's syndrome, and probably to other postinfectious arthropathies.

Induction of autoantibodies.   The appearance of autoantibodies during infection is well recognized; examples include cold agglutinins in *Mycoplasma pneumoniae* infection, haemolysins in infectious mononucleosis, and anti-A blood group antibodies in type 14 pneumococcal infections. Cross-reactions between human and microbial antigens have occasionally been demonstrated. Antibodies to cardiac muscle can be found in some patients with *Strep. pyogenes* infection, and lymphocytes activated by *Klebsiella* antigens will also attack HLA B27 tissue type antigens.

It is also possible that the infectious process can modify or damage some human antigens so that antibodies will be mobilized against them.

The formation of immune complexes.   These are envisaged as soluble antigen–antibody complexes which may be deposited in tissues under certain circumstances. They are demonstrable in the circulation and in the skin, synovial membranes and glomerular basement membranes of patients with inflammatory and autoimmune disorders.

Immune complexes circulate in the serum of patients with both rheumatic fever and poststreptococcal nephritis and are associated in the former case with high, and the latter case low, levels of complement. They are also demonstrable in the synovial fluid of some patients with postinfectious arthritis.

Further evidence that certain disorders are associated with soluble substances is available in their prompt response to plasma exchange. This is seen in some patients with postinfectious polyneuritis.

Persisting low-grade infection.   This is difficult to separate from the acute infectious state. Antibodies of IgM type persist for many weeks after acute viral hepatitis, infectious mononucleosis and toxoplasmosis, diseases which are often followed by prolonged debility. Whether this indicates prolonged infection or a persisting immune reaction is not yet clear.

The effect, if any, of latent virus infection which appears to involve no immune response, is a matter for speculation. It is known that several viruses can exist in human tissues without ill effect. These viruses may have a pathogenic role if the immune system is disturbed by disease.

Rheumatic fever

Epidemiology
This syndrome appears in up to 3% of patients with clinically evident
Streptococcus pyogenes tonsillitis. It does not occur after streptococcal
skin infection. Attacks are most likely in patients between the ages of 5
and 17 years, with severe tonsillitis, and with a history of previous
rheumatic fever. The usual interval between tonsillitis and rheumatic
fever is 2–3 weeks.

Clinical features
These are present in various combinations of five major manifestations
and several minor manifestations which together comprise Jones' criteria
for the diagnosis of rheumatic fever. The most common presenting complaints are fever and arthritis.

Major manifestations	*Minor manifestations*
Arthritis	Fever
Carditis	Previous episodes
Chorea	Raised ESR/C-reactive protein
Rash	Cardiographic abnormalities
Nodules	Arthralgia

If there is evidence of recent *Strep. pyogenes* infection two major, or
one major and two minor criteria, are strong evidence for a positive
diagnosis. A florid clinical picture is rarely seen nowadays in developed
countries, but still appears where overcrowding is common and medical
treatment of the original infection is difficult to deliver.

Arthritis.   This is typically described as 'flitting, large-joint arthritis'.
The most-affected joints are the knees, ankles, wrists and elbows. Pain,
swelling and redness may appear suddenly only to subside after a few
days and appear elsewhere, frequently in the opposite joint.

Carditis.   This is a pancarditis, affecting the pericardium and myocardium as well as the endocardium.
 The pericarditis is acute and exudative. It is clinically apparent with
pain and friction rub in the more severe cases. Large pericardial effusions, however, are rare.
 Myocarditis varies greatly in severity, in some cases producing only
minor cardiographic abnormalities or first-degree heart block, in others
causing severe dysrrhythmias and heart failure.
 Endocarditis is almost always left-sided, mostly affecting the mitral
valve, though the aortic valve may be involved especially in boys. Signs
include softening of the first heart sound, the appearance of a third heart

sound and of mid-systolic or mid-diastolic (Carey–Coombs) murmurs. With recurrent attacks the chordae tendinae become shortened, causing regurgitation, and the cusps stick together causing stenosis. Severe fibrosis, calcification and immobilization of the valve can eventually take place.

Caution.   The clinical signs of heart failure can be very subtle in small children. Pulmonary congestion may produce a cough giving a false impression of respiratory disease and hepatic distension may cause vague epigastric pain.

Care must also be taken not to confuse bacterial endocarditis with recurrent rheumatic fever. Blood cultures should always be obtained, and serological tests for unusual infections may also be indicated in doubtful cases.

Chorea.   This occurs in about 5% of patients, particularly girls in the higher age groups. The frequent, purposeless, involuntary movements may be dismissed as nervous tics, and the patient often attempts to conceal them.

Rash.   This is usually erythema marginatum. Large raised crescentic and serpiginous lesions appear on the trunk and thighs. The rash may be fleeting and appear only during peaks of fever.

Rheumatic nodules.   These are seen in under 5% of patients and often coincide with severe carditis. They may be up to a centimetre or more in diameter, appearing on the extensor surfaces usually near large joints.

Diagnosis

Demonstration of recent Strep. pyogenes *infection.*   Throat swabs will produce positive cultures in a number of patients who are still infected or who have become carriers. Failing this, significant antistreptolysin O titres (ASOT) should be sought in paired sera. A single elevated titre is better evidence than nothing if paired sera are not obtainable. In the small proportion of patients with normal ASOT (below 200 u/ml) other antibodies, such as anti DNAase B can be estimated.

Evidence of rheumatic disease.   Frequent examination of the patient, coupled with cardiography and estimation of the erythrocyte sedimentation rate, should eventually reveal an adequate combination of criteria to permit diagnosis.

Biopsy of affected tissue will occasionally aid diagnosis. Typical foci of inflammation (Aschoff bodies) may be seen on microscopy.

Treatment

Eradicate the streptococci.   This is best achieved with a 7–10 days' course of intramuscular benzylpenicillin. Oral penicillins may not be successful.

Treat the inflammatory lesions. The drug of choice for this is aspirin which may be given in the maximum tolerated dose. Other non-steroidal anti-inflammatory agents (NSAID) may be helpful if aspirin is not tolerated. Corticosteroids do not appear to influence the course of the disease. Bedrest is advisable while there is evidence of active carditis.

Prevention
Further attacks of streptococcal tonsillitis can be prevented by prophylactic penicillin treatment. A useful regimen is intramuscular benzathine penicillin 1.2 mega units monthly. Oral penicillin V 125–250 mg twice daily, or sulphadiazine 0.5–1.0 mg daily are acceptable alternatives.

It is usual to continue prophylaxis until a child leaves school. Those who later work in schools or hospitals, or attend college may continue prophylaxis for longer, as may those with evidence of severe carditis. The risk of further attacks is much reduced after the age of 30 years.

Reiter's syndrome

Epidemiology
This is a rare condition which usually affects men, appearing 10–14 days after the onset of non-specific urethritis (NSU). It occasionally complicates bacillary dysentery, when it can affect either sex. Patients are almost always of tissue type HLA B27.

Clinical features
The major features are conjunctivitis, synovitis and mucocutaneous rash. The synovitis affects large joints, particularly knees, ankles and shoulders causing pain and effusion. Small joints and tendon sheaths may also be involved with surrounding redness and oedema. Sacroiliitis may occur.

The typical rash is circinate balanitis, consisting of roughly circular weepy lesions with crusted or flaking margins. Whitish patches may appear in the mouth. A later skin eruption, keratoderma blenorrhagica, often appears on the palms and soles. These lesions are heaped up, brownish and keratotic with scattered flat vesicles.

Rare manifestations include aortitis, aortic incompetence, cardiac dysrrhythmias and uveitis. Relapses and recurrences are common, giving the illness a prolonged, fluctuating course.

Diagnosis
Confirm the diagnosis of urethritis. Mucous threads will be seen in the first-glass urine. Pus cells are present in smears of urethral scrapings.

Gonococci should not be seen unless the two conditions coexist. Some laboratories may be able to isolate chlamydiae from urethral swabs.

The coincidence of typical clinical features with urethritis is diagnostic.

Treatment
Eradicate the urethral infection.   This can usually be achieved with a 3-week course of oral tetracycline or erythromycin.

Treat the inflammatory condition.   Non-steroidal anti-inflammatory drugs (NSAID) such as aspirin, phenylbutazone or ibuprofen are the drugs of choice. Corticosteroids are rarely useful. Relapses should be treated in the same way as the acute illness.

Poststreptococcal glomerulonephritis

Epidemiology
This disorder can be a sequel to *Streptococcus pyogenes* infection of the skin or throat. It has particularly been associated with *Strep. pyogenes* M-types 12, 4 and 25. The glomerulonephritis begins 1–4 weeks after the acute infection, ususally 10–14 days, and is most common in children between the ages of 1 – 5 years.

Clinical features
The onset is rapid with malaise, anorexia and slight fever. The child's mother usually notices haematuria, oliguria and puffiness of the child's eyelids. There may also be loin pain, headache and oedema of the feet and hands.

The haematuria is seldom gross, the urine being smoky or pinkish in most cases; occasionally it is only detectable on microscopy. Proteinuria is likewise mild and rarely results in significant loss of body protein.

Most patients have an elevated blood pressure during the acute illness, with diastolic measurements of 90–100 mmHg.

The natural course of the disease is short. The oliguria improves and diuresis often occurs within a week, though complete recovery can take place after up to a month of oliguria. Mild impairment of creatinine clearance and microscopic haematuria may persist for several weeks. About 5% of patients, however, fail to make a complete recovery. They may remain asymptomatic for many years, but have increasing proteinuria and haematuria eventually ending in chronic renal failure. A further 1 or 2% have life-threatening disease with uraemia, hyperkalaemia or hypertensive encephalopathy.

Diagnosis
Demonstration of recent Strep. pyogenes *infection.*   Culture of throat or

skin swabs, or rising ASOT and anti DNAase B titres will usually provide adequate evidence.

Urine examination.   Chemical testing and microscopy will confirm proteinuria and haematuria. Epithelial casts are seen on microscopy, and red blood cells mixed with the epithelial cells confirm the glomerular origin of the bleeding.

Renal biopsy.   This is rarely carried out in uncomplicated cases. It shows an acute exudative glomerulonephritis, with many enlarged glomeruli, proliferation of endothelial cells and infiltration by neutrophils. Immunofluorescent staining or electronmicroscopy shows irregular deposits of immune complexes on the glomerular basement membrane.

Caution.   Transient haematuria is quite common during acute *Strep. pyogenes* infections. It does not mean that glomerulonephritis will necessarily follow.

Glomerulonephritis of various types and severity can occur rarely in infections other than those due to *Strep. pyogenes*. Atypical pneumonias, staphylococcal infections and malignant malaria can all cause significant renal lesions. First-generation cephalosporins, methicillin, aminoglycosides and other antibiotics can also affect renal function and confuse the clinical picture, even to the extent of causing cells and casts to appear in the urine.

Treatment
Treat the streptococcal infection.   Throat infections often require treatment with intramuscular benzylpenicillin. Superficial skin infections may be treated with oral penicillins (see Chapters 2 and 3). Prophylaxis against further attacks is not required.

The renal lesion.   This usually recovers without specific treatment. The few patients with severe disease may require dietary protein and potassium restriction, ion exchange resins or even peritoneal dialysis. Diuretics can be used to treat oedema and to encourage urine output.

Specialist advice and renal biopsy are required in the rare cases who fail to recover.

Henoch–Schönlein syndrome

Epidemiology
The postinfectious nature of this disorder is not well established. Although cases have been recorded after streptococcal and other upper respiratory infections and after typhoid immunization, many patients cannot remember any preceding illness.

Those most commonly affected are schoolchildren and teenagers, but adult cases are occasionally seen.

Clinical features

These are skin rash, abdominal pain, synovitis and glomerulonephritis.

The rash is due to vasculitis. It consists of weals or papules which are often itchy or painful and which usually develop petechial and purpuric elements. Small haemorrhagic bullae may also develop. The thighs, buttocks and lower legs are most often affected.

The abdominal pain is caused by vasculitic lesions in the bowel wall. The lesions are surrounded by serosanguineous swellings, and large swellings of the mucosa can lead to intussusception, a recognized hazard in children.

The synovitis often causes large-joint pain and effusion, especially in the knees and ankles. Tendon sheath involvement may produce redness and oedema of the dorsa of the hands or feet.

Glomerulonephritis affects about a third of the child cases and probably a greater proportion of adults. In children transient haematuria and proteinuria may be the only abnormality. Adults, however, may develop progressive renal disease.

The acute attack may last for up to 6 weeks; a fluctuating course is common and late relapses sometimes occur.

Diagnosis

The clinical features are distinct, though non-purpuric rashes sometimes cause confusion.

There is often a moderate leukocytosis and sometimes an eosinophilia. The erythrocyte sedimentation rate is raised.

If renal biopsy is performed it reveals a focal proliferative glomerulonephritis quite different from the lesion of poststreptococcal nephritis.

Treatment

Most cases recover spontaneously without intervention. Aspirin and other anti-inflammatory drugs help to reduce joint pain. Corticosteroids have little influence on the course of the disease.

Glomerulonephritis in adults is often a serious problem. It requires expert assessment and may need vigorous treatment with corticosteroids and other drugs. The response to treatment may be disappointing.

Erythema multiforme

Epidemiology

This is a skin disorder which mainly affects teenagers and young adults. It can occur after streptococcal infections, herpes simplex and atypical pneumonias. It has also been associated with long-acting penicillins, sulphonamides and other antibiotics.

Clinical features

The patient usually presents with a rash and fever. The rash consists of

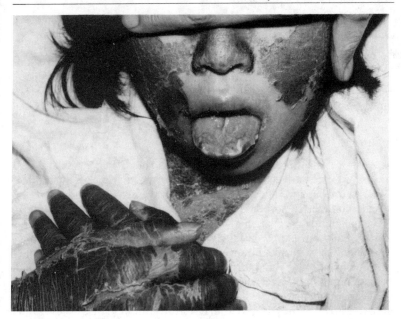

Fig. 27. Stevens–Johnson syndrome: mucosal lesions and desquamation of skin.

typical 'iris lesions', raised discoid lesions with purple or necrotic centres. There may also be a rash of many-shaped pink papules, resembling confetti. The extent of the rash can vary greatly, but the palms, soles and face are usually affected. Bullae may develop in severe rashes, and if these are extensive they may break, leaving large denuded areas. This process is called toxic epidermal necrolysis.

Stevens–Johnson syndrome. In severe cases the mucous membranes are also affected. The mouth is particularly susceptible (Fig. 27), but the conjunctivae and genital mucosae can also be involved. Severe Stevens–Johnson syndrome can be life-threatening, as heat, fluids, protein and electrolytes are lost from the skin, and bacterial pathogens can easily invade the denuded areas.

Diagnosis
The clinical picture is distinct. The erythrocyte sedimentation rate is usually very high.

Treatment
Most of the milder cases resolve spontaneously within 2–3 weeks. The rash heals by staining and desquamation.

Severe cases can often be terminated by corticosteroid treatment. A typical course would be prednisolone 60 mg daily for 5 days, followed by gradually reducing doses.

Caution   Blood cultures should be taken frequently while skin defects persist, as bacteraemia easily occurs and may be masked by steroid therapy.

Aesthenic states

Not all postinfectious disorders are well defined. Vague malaise and excessive fatigue are common complaints, particularly after such infections as viral hepatitis and infectious mononucleosis. Laboratory tests are usually completely normal and recovery occurs in a matter of weeks.

A small minority of patients suffer severe and prolonged debility of this kind, usually after apparently trivial respiratory infections which were assumed to have been of viral aetiology. A distinct feature of the debility is the conviction of the patient that no improvement is occurring. All possible laboratory investigations remain obstinately normal except for occasional evidence of recent viral infection, or minor electromyographic abnormalities. Some patients undergo fruitless psychiatric investigation because of their apparently groundless complaints. Fortunately, gradual improvement takes place in a number of cases, even after as long as 2 years of disability.

Recent investigations have shown that a proportion of those patients may have an acquired abnormality of muscle metabolism. If this can be confirmed, the study of postinfectious disorders may afford a new approach to the understanding of infection and the pathogenesis of infectious disease; much remains to be learned in these fields.

Further reading

CHRISTIE, A.B. (1980) *Infectious Diseases: Epidemiology and Clinical Practice*, 3rd ed. Edinburgh: Churchill Livingstone.

GRIECO, M.H. (ed.) (1980) *Infections in the Abnormal Host*. New York: Yorke Medical Books.

MANDEL, G.L., DOUGLAS, R.G. and BENNET, J.E. (1979) *Principles and Practice of Infectious Diseases*. New York: John Wiley and Sons Inc.

MANSON-BAHR, P.E.C. and APTED, F.I.C. (1982) *Manson's Tropical Diseases*, 18th ed. London: Baillière Tindall.

TOPLEY, W.W.C. and WILSON, G.S. (1975) *Principles of Bacteriology and Immunity*, 6th ed. London: Edward Arnold (Publishers) Ltd.

Index